T0323424

Conceiving People

Conceiving People

*Genetic Knowledge and the Ethics of
Sperm and Egg Donation*

DANIEL GROLL

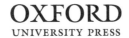

OXFORD
UNIVERSITY PRESS

Oxford University Press is a department of the University of Oxford. It furthers
the University's objective of excellence in research, scholarship, and education
by publishing worldwide. Oxford is a registered trade mark of Oxford University
Press in the UK and certain other countries.

Published in the United States of America by Oxford University Press
198 Madison Avenue, New York, NY 10016, United States of America.

Library of Congress Control Number: 2021911837
ISBN 978–0–19–006305–4

DOI: 10.1093/oso/9780190063054.001.0001

1 3 5 7 9 8 6 4 2

Printed by Integrated Books International, United States of America

For Aub and Lu

Contents

Acknowledgments

In August 2017, I was walking in Holyrood Park with Tom, an old pal from graduate school. I was recently tenured and Tom was just about to come up (reader: he got it). While walking under the Salisbury Crags, we reflected on our work to that point in our careers. We both agreed that neither of us had a book in us. After our walk, we met up with Jenn—another old pal from grad school—who asked me what I was working on. I told them about a paper I had just started about the ethics of anonymous gamete donation. As the conversation got going—about the nature of parenthood, about why people care about their genetic lineage, about why people donate their gametes—it became clear to me that everything I wanted to say was too big for a single paper. By the end of the evening, I realized I had a book in me. Now it is out of me and in your hands ... which sounds grosser than I intend.

I am profoundly grateful to the many people who have helped me to write this book. A good portion of my thinking on these matters has been formed in dialogue with the fabulous students I get to teach every year at Carleton College in my "Family Values" first-year seminar. The heart of the book was conceived and written during my yearlong sabbatical as a visitor in the Philosophy Department at the University of Edinburgh with the support of a generous grant from the Bruce Carroll Memorial Fund. I could not have asked for a better setting in which to work on this project. Special thanks go to Guy Fletcher, Philip Cook, and Sarah Chan for inviting me to participate in the Ethics Workshop, the Political Theory Research Group, and the Mason Institute Work-in-Progress group, respectively. Debbie Roberts and, once again, Guy Fletcher were constant companions—philosophical and otherwise—during my time in Edinburgh. I love talking to them about my work and theirs, and I look forward to welcoming them for their sabbatical to Northfield, Minnesota.

I am grateful to audiences at Warwick University and Umeå University as well as to Thomas Lockhart, Kalle Grill, Anca Gheuas, Jason Hanna, and anonymous reviewers for Oxford University Press (OUP) and the *Journal of Medicine and Philosophy* for providing valuable feedback on draft chapters. Thanks as well to Walter Martin for permission to use a verse from his song *Hey Sister!* in chapter 4 and the *Journal of Medicine and Philosophy* for allowing me to include material from my paper "Well-Being, Gamete Donation, and Genetic Knowledge: The Significant Interest View" in chapter 3. Jason Decker is my go-to philosophy conversation partner and has discussed many of the ideas in this book over many a pint of high quality beer (for him) and low quality beer (for me). Micah Lott and Jenn Lockhart have been fantastic writing partners these past few years and gave characteristically excellent comments on multiple chapters. Ben Richardson read the entire final draft of the manuscript, catching numerous errors and offering very helpful substantive comments along the way.

I also benefited tremendously from two workshops devoted to the manuscript. The first, held at Oxford in May 2017 and organized by Jonathan Parry and Jessica Begon, brought together Liam Shields, Hallvard Lillehammer, Tim Fowler, and Anna Smajdor to offer comments on early drafts of three chapters. The second, held over Zoom in June 2020 and organized by Alice MacLachlan, brought together Alice, Carolyn McLeod, Samantha Brennan, Olivia Schumann, Andrée-Anne Cormier, and Emily Tilton to discuss a complete draft of the book. The final product was greatly improved by their feedback, with substantial parts of chapters 5 and 8 being utterly transformed for the better. The work required to complete the book was supported by the Hewlett Mellon & Dean's Fellowship at Carleton College.

Susan Golombok, Wes Markofski, Liz Raleigh, and Douglas NeJaime passed along very helpful sources in response to my questions about the sociology and law of new family forms. Kim Decker helped me figure out how to decipher case law references. Kaethe Schwehn provided the hilarious list of common lies parents tell their children in chapter 2. John Appleby, who has considerably more expertise on philosophical issues in reproductive medicine than I do, provided excellent advice, various helpful resources, and a much-needed dose of encouragement at a key moment in the manuscript's life. Ned Hall generously answered some questions I had about how to think about causal contribution of genetics to phenotypical traits.

A few people deserve more robust "Thanks." Lisa Fedorak did a fabulous job putting together the index. Lucy Randall and Hannah Doyle at OUP helped a newbie navigate the process of writing a book, patiently answering questions I've been asking from the fall of 2017 to literally just a few minutes ago about various aspects of the book publishing process.

Kim Brownlee generously shared her book proposals with me to serve as a template for my own and then offered extremely helpful feedback on a draft of my proposal. She also passed on her tremendously useful advice for writing, without which I probably would never have finished the book: "Write every day. Stop when it's no longer fun."

Rivka Weinberg read and commented on multiple drafts of multiple chapters. She also provided a model of philosophical writing, in the form of her own book, which gave me something to aspire to. Rivka's writing makes me think and it makes me laugh, not infrequently at the same time. When trying to figure out how to formulate an idea, I often ask myself the question "WWRW?" ("What Would Rivka Write?").

Dorothy MacKinnon is an extraordinary copy editor who has saved me countless painful hours of reading my own work and improved my writing along the way. She deserves a prize, which will come in the form of a complimentary book about the ethics of gamete donation.

Alice MacLachlan deserves special mention. Alice and I started talking philosophy in her dorm room at Pearson College in 1996 and haven't stopped since. Alice's fingerprints are on every idea in this book (including those she disagrees with). Alice read early drafts. Alice read late drafts. Portions of long text chains about bionormativity, parenting, gender, and genetic relatedness have been imported, whole cloth, into this book. Alice also very kindly let me choose a title for the book that is close to the title of her paper, "Conceiving Differently." This book would look very different without her contributions.

I also want to thank Dan Hernandez. He didn't actually do anything. But he has a good streak of being mentioned in the acknowledgments of friends' books and I don't want to break it.

I do *not* want to thank my children. Minutes after learning OUP gave me a contract, I picked up my then five-year-old son from school. On the drive home, I sighed loudly and said "Oh boy."

"Why did you say "Oh boy?" my son asked.

"Well, I just found out the publisher wants to publish my book, which is exciting. But now it's hitting me that I really need to write the whole thing and that's stressful. But I can do it."

I suggested we start up a chant of "Dad, you can do it! Dad, you can do it!" But, sensing an opportunity to aggravate me, he immediately started chanting, "Dad can't do it! Dad can't do it!" Then, in case the knife wasn't in far enough, he started chanting, "It is too hard! It is too hard!"

As for my eleven-year-old daughter, we had the following exchange about the book this summer:

"Are you still writing your book?"
"Yes I am."
"Really? I would have given up by now."

By way of revenge, let me reveal a secret in these pages knowing that my kids are unlikely to read them for many years, if at all. In February 2020, in the depths of Minnesota winter, when it looked like we might all be locked down for a good long time, we decided to buy a Nintendo Switch for the children just in case we found ourselves cooped up together for weeks or even months on end. The plan was to bring out the Switch only if things got desperate (not out of any sense of parenting virtue, but to avoid having to put the genie back in the bottle post-pandemic). The Switch is still sitting in the closet, untouched. The children live in total ignorance of its existence. Until now. THERE WAS A NINTENDO SWITCH IN THE CLOSET CHILDREN! YOU HAD NO IDEA! Also, I love you both very much.

Finally: Emily Carroll. The original draft of this acknowledgment had a loving paragraph right here about all the help and encouragement you've provided me while writing the book. I sent it to you. You wrote back with one word: "BORING." And then you encouraged me to say something about farts. And then you said: "I'm too lowbrow for dedications. I didn't even put in any in my Doctorate of Nursing Practice Thesis. NONE. I didn't thank any of you fools." Well, this fool thanks you.

1

Introduction

The Central Question

Here is a picture of my parents:

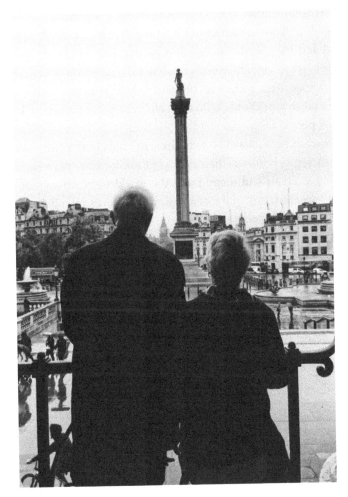

The author's parents

Conceiving People. Daniel Groll, Oxford University Press. © Oxford University Press 2021.
DOI: 10.1093/oso/9780190063054.003.0001

What does it mean to you when I say, "These are my parents"? What would you want to know in order to figure out whether they are, in fact, my parents? Whether they are my genetic progenitors? Whether the woman on the right gestated me? Whether they raised me?

We all know that the relationships captured by these questions—the genetic relationship, the gestational relationship, and the social relationship—can come apart. Some children's social parents are also their genetic parents, though they were gestated by someone to whom they bear no genetic relation. Some children's social parents are neither their genetic nor their gestational parents. Some children are genetically related to, and gestated by, one of their social parents but not the other. And some children were gestated by one social parent, but are genetically related only to the other.

This book is about the ethics of intentionally creating children for whom the social and the genetic relationship are separate, either altogether or in part. This is what happens when children are created via *donor conception*. In donor conception, someone "donates"[1] their gametes—either sperm or eggs—to a person, or people, who want children but require genetic material from other people.

Each year, tens of thousands of children are conceived with donated sperm or eggs.[2] By some estimates, there are over 1 million donor-conceived people in the United States and many more the world over. Anonymous gamete donation—where the identity of the donor is never intended to be made available to the donor-conceived person—is prohibited in places like the UK and Sweden. In these countries, donor-conceived people may learn the identity of their donor when they turn 18. In other countries, such as the United States and Canada, anonymous gamete donation is not only allowed, but also widely practiced.[3] The children created from anonymously donated gametes may never know who one of their genetic parents is.[4]

Is this a problem? If so, why? And if not, why not? These questions are profoundly important to the millions of people who are part of the donor conception community. This community includes not just donor-conceived

---

[1] This term is not entirely apt for reasons I'll come to soon.

[2] Most commonly donated sperm, less commonly donated eggs, and even less commonly donated sperm and eggs, i.e. "double donation."

[3] For a helpful table that shows the current rules surrounding gamete donation in various countries, see Ariana Eunjung Cha, "Her 44 Siblings Were Conceived with One Donor's Sperm: Here's How It Was Possible," *Washington Post*, September 12, 2018, https://www.washingtonpost.com/graphics/2018/health/44-donor-siblings-and-counting/.

[4] Or parents in the case of double donation.

people, but also their parents, gamete donors, and an entire segment of the fertility industry that acquires and provides donated gametes to intended parents, often for profit.

But the ethical significance of conceiving children with donated gametes extends well beyond the donor conception community. You cannot think about the ethics of donor conception without confronting questions that matter to everyone: What is the significance of genetic relatedness? What makes someone a parent? What obligations do parents have to their children?

These questions matter to you even if your family situation—as a child or a parent—is utterly stereotypical, conforming to the "traditional" conception of the family as consisting of a mother, a father, and children that are genetic offspring. Everyone has views—however implicit—about what it means to be a parent, about the nature of family-relatedness, about what kinds of things parents should (and should not) do for their children. You might well go through life without ever thinking about, let alone forming views on, the pros and cons of using flatwound strings on an electric guitar. But it is impossible to navigate our world, given the kinds of creatures we are, without having some views about the nature of parents and families, even if they never come to the surface for critical scrutiny. The practice of donor conception provides a vivid occasion to think about the nature of the relationships that are a central part of everybody's life.

1. What this book is and isn't about

Donor conception has changed a lot in the past 60 years or so. Back in the "bad old days," donor conception was something of an *ad hoc* affair: a couple (and it was always a heterosexual couple) who could not conceive on their own would find a doctor who would secure donor gametes for insemination. Sometimes those gametes came from the doctor himself.[5] Sometimes it was from a friend

---

[5] And, indeed, this still happens with shocking frequency. The big difference these days is that the doctors are doing something entirely deceptive and illegal since the intended parents believe the gametes are coming from a donor they have chosen. See *CBC News*, "Fertility Doctor Implanted Own Sperm in Clients 11 Times, Lawsuit Alleges," April 5, 2018, https://www.cbc.ca/news/canada/ottawa/fertility-doctor-own-sperm-11-times-1.4606814; Jacqueline Mroz, "Their Mothers Chose Donor Sperm: The Doctors Used Their Own," *New York Times*, August 21, 2019, https://www.nytimes.com/2019/08/21/health/sperm-donors-fraud-doctors.html; Christopher F. Schuetze, "Dutch Fertility Doctor Swapped Donors' Sperm with His, Lawsuit Claims," *New York Times*, May 15, 2017, https://www.nytimes.com/2017/05/15/world/europe/dutch-fertility-doctor-swapped-donors-sperm-with-his-lawsuit-claims.html.

or acquaintance. The intended parents basically had no choices when it came to who their donor was and little or no descriptive information about him[6]—what he looked like, his level of education, his medical history, *etc.* Donor conception was essentially "off the books." The law didn't recognize the possibility of someone donating gametes but having no legal rights or responsibilities with respect to the resulting child, and so records were either not kept in the first place or not kept for very long. The donor was assured anonymity in the sense that it was simply understood that his identity would never be discovered.

Typical donor conception looks very different today. It usually involves as least two transactions.[7] When it comes to conceiving with donated sperm, a sperm bank first acquires sperm from a donor (in the United States, for example, donors are paid; in Canada they are not). Second, that sperm is sold to (an) intended parent(s) who can either use the sperm themselves without a fertility clinic[8] or do *in vitro* fertilization through a fertility clinic. According to Naomi Cahn, there are currently more than 150 sperm banks in the United States and "they can ship frozen sperm anywhere."[9] A vial of sperm can cost as little as $350.

Egg donation is a different kettle of fish. As Cahn notes:

> Buying donor eggs is more difficult, and more expensive. Until recently, there were relatively few egg brokers, and eggs had to be fresh. With new technology allowing for the successful freezing of eggs, and with increasing demand, there are growing numbers of egg sellers. But, unlike sperm, donor eggs require the use of a fertility clinic and a cycle of in vitro fertilization.[10]

Intended parents have a lot of options when it comes to choosing a donor. They can filter donors by race, education level, eye color, hair color, or hobbies. The California Cryobank allows you to choose donors on the basis of their resemblance to celebrities like Ben Affleck or Brett Favre.[11]

---

[6] And it was always a "him." Egg donation only became possible in the 1980s.

[7] Naomi R. Cahn, *The New Kinship: Constructing Donor-Conceived Families* (New York: NYU Press, 2013), 44.

[8] By using what is known as the Turkey Baster Method. CoParents, "Artificial Insemination: The Turkey Baster Method," accessed August 2, 2020, https://www.coparents.com/blog/the-turkey-baster-method-what-is-it-and-how-to-perform-it/.

[9] Cahn, *The New Kinship*, 19.

[10] Cahn, *The New Kinship*, 19.

[11] From Cahn: "Through the trademarked 'CCB Donor Look-a-Likes' program, prospective purchasers can click on a link that will take them to photos of two or three celebrities whom the staff has decided are the closest matches to the donor." Cahn, *The New Kinship*, 52.

Offering intended parents these kinds of choices raises serious questions about donor conception: Is it ethical for people to buy and sell gametes in the first place? What kind of medical screening should be in place for potential donors? How many offspring should it be permissible to create from one donor? To what extent should intended parents have a say about the genetic features of the donor they choose? What does it even mean for donated gametes to have a "race," and how does the practice of "racing" gametes connect to, and further entrench, problematic notions of race, kinship, and relatedness?[12]

These are all important questions. But I don't address them in this book. Instead, my focus is on what I will call *the central question* that confronts many people who plan to conceive with donated gametes, namely: Should they use an anonymous donor or not?

Of course, calling this *the central question* presumes that conceiving children with donated gametes is permissible in the first place. Not everyone thinks it is. Anti-natalists think that all procreation is impermissible and so will object to donor conception just because it is a form of procreation. I do not take on anti-natalist arguments at all in this book.[13]

But there are others who, while not opposed to procreation in general, are opposed to donor conception because of how it relates (problematically in their view) to parental responsibility[14] or healthy identity-determination.[15] I *do* discuss those views in this book. But I do not attempt to first show that donor conception is permissible and only then turn to the *central question*. Rather, my responses to these kinds of views emerge in my answers to the *central question*.

My project, then, begins *in medias res*: it proceeds from the fact that donor conception is, and will continue to be, widely practiced. And it turns an

---

[12] Camisha A. Russell, *The Assisted Reproduction of Race* (Bloomington: Indiana University Press, 2018).

[13] There is a distinction between what we might call "in-principle anti-natalists" and "in-practice anti-natalists." In-principle anti-natalists, like David Benatar and Seana Shiffrin, object to procreation as such because of its intrinsic structural features (though Shiffrin's brand of anti-natalism is less demanding, I think, than Benatar's). In-practice anti-natalists object to procreation given contingent facts about the world (such as, for instance, the fact that there are many existing children that need parents). See Tina Rulli, "Preferring a Genetically-Related Child," *Journal of Moral Philosophy* 13, no. 6 (2016): 669–98; David Benatar, *Better Never to Have Been: The Harm of Coming into Existence* (Oxford: Oxford University Press, 2008); Seana Valentine Shiffrin, "Wrongful Life, Procreative Responsibility, and the Significance of Harm," *Legal Theory* 5, no. 2 (1999): 117–48.

[14] Rivka Weinberg, *The Risk of a Lifetime: How, When, and Why Procreation May Be Permissible* (New York: Oxford University Press, 2016), chapter 2.

[15] J. David Velleman, "The Gift of Life," *Philosophy & Public Affairs* 36, no. 3 (2008): 245–66; J. David Velleman, "Family History," *Philosophical Papers* 34, no. 3 (2005): 357–78.

interrogative eye on how it should proceed with respect to the issue of donor anonymity.

2. Getting clear on terms

My answer to the central question is this: intended parents who plan to conceive with donated gametes should, generally speaking, use a donor whose identity will be made available to the resulting child. This is, roughly, because doing so puts their child in a good position to satisfy the child's likely future interest in knowing who their donor is. I say more about how this argument unfolds later in the chapter. For now, though, I want to explain how I'll be using five key terms that appear throughout the book: "donor," "genetic knowledge," "anonymous donor," "open donor," and "known donor."

2.1. Donor

Before discussing the different kinds of gamete donors, I want to highlight how inapt the term "donor" is to describe many people who provide gametes to others. As we've already seen, many donors (like those in the United States) are paid for their services. When someone is compensated for providing some good, we don't usually say they've donated it. There are interesting and important questions about why gamete providers are usually called "donors" rather than, for example, "sellers."[16] Nonetheless, I stick with the language of "donors" for two reasons.

First, there really are gamete *donors*, people who provide gametes for no compensation. I could distinguish these (genuine) donors from the sellers. Alternatively, I could use the term "gamete providers," but I worry that this would make people think of sperm and egg *clinics* rather than the people providing their gametes. This leads me to my second reason for sticking with the term "donor": it is so widespread that I fear using any other term will just invite confusion, particularly given that basically all my sources use the term. So: "donor" it is.

---

[16] Cahn remarks that the "donor world is characterized by a vocabulary that serves as a cultural clue (and cue) to our interpretation and understanding of these new families." Cahn, *The New Kinship*, 7.

2.2. Genetic knowledge

People who carry the BRCA 1 or 2 gene mutation are highly susceptible to developing breast cancer. Suppose you learn that you have the mutation. You have learned something about your genetic makeup. It makes a lot of sense to call the kind of knowledge you have acquired "genetic knowledge." Someone who has his entire genome sequenced (and is in a position to understand the results) has a *lot* of genetic knowledge.

This is not how I will use the term "genetic knowledge." When I talk about "genetic knowledge" I mean to refer to knowledge of who one's genetic progenitors are. In other words, the person who is seeking genetic knowledge, as I shall use the term, wants to know who her genetic parents are. Now, what it means to know who someone is—i.e. their identity—is a thornier issue than it appears. Knowing a person's name isn't enough. And sometimes, neither is knowing a lot about a person or even being acquainted with them ("I just had a great conversation with someone, but I don't know who he is!"). Conversely, you can know who someone is without knowing much of anything about them or without ever having met them.

My guess is that the variety of ways we talk about "knowing who someone is" is not amenable to a unified account. But for my purposes we can rely on an intuitive conception of what it means for a donor-conceived person to know who her donor is. Someone who knows her donor only by the donor number does not know who her donor is (even if she has a decent amount of information *about* the donor). Contrariwise, someone who knows her donor's name and has enough information to fairly reliably pick him out or track him down knows who her donor is. This person could, as it were, point to the donor were he in front of her and say, "That's him." This person has genetic knowledge as I shall be using the term.

Notice that my conception of having genetic knowledge falls short of another way we might understand what it means to know who one's genetic parents are: having a relationship with them or, more minimally, being acquainted with them.[17] Someone could have genetic knowledge as I use the term without ever meeting their donor.

---

[17] This is the kind of genetic knowledge that really matters for Velleman. Velleman, "Family History."

So we have three senses of "genetic knowledge" on the table (with my usage in boldface):[18]

1. Medical genetic knowledge: knowledge of one's genome, particular genetic traits, *etc.* (in the language of genomics).
2. **Progenitor genetic knowledge: knowledge of who one's genetic progenitors are.**
3. Relationship genetic knowledge: being in a relationship with one's genetic parents.

My focus in this book is on the second kind of genetic knowledge. I will argue that intended parents should put their donor-conceived child in a position to acquire genetic knowledge. In other words, they should put their child in a position to know *who* their genetic progenitor is.

There are connections between the three kinds of genetic knowledge I've identified. Someone might want progenitor genetic knowledge or relationship genetic knowledge as a means of gaining valuable medical genetic knowledge. Or someone might want medical genetic knowledge as a means of gaining progenitor genetic knowledge, which, in turn, they might want in order to gain relationship genetic knowledge.

In light of these possible connections, you might think this: a plausible account of why intended parents should put their child in a position to acquire progenitor genetic knowledge will appeal to the value of having medical genetic knowledge or relationship genetic knowledge (or both). But that's just not true. Donor-conceived people's interest in acquiring progenitor genetic knowledge (when they have such an interest—not all do) usually goes well beyond an interest in having medical genetic knowledge, but usually falls short of an interest in relationship genetic knowledge. What they usually

---

[18] There is a fourth kind of genetic knowledge, what I will call *ancestral* genetic knowledge, i.e. knowledge of one's genetic ancestors. I say a little more about it, and why I will not be talking about it, presently. My three categories of genetic knowledge basically come from Vardit Ravitsky, "Knowing Where You Come From: The Rights of Donor-Conceived Individuals and the Meaning of Genetic Relatedness," *Minnesota Journal of Law, Science & Technology* 11 (2010): 665. She refers to them as different "aspects" of the right to know one's genetic origins: the medical aspect, the identity aspect, and the relational aspect (668). My categories depart a little from Ravitsky's. Her "aspects" encompass the *kind* of knowledge being sought along with the *reason* for seeking it (e.g. "The *identity aspect* points towards the right to **personal information about the donor as a person** (narrative information) **that would assist offspring in overcoming identity issues**" (668, boldface added), whereas mine only include the former. Ravitsky also identifies a fourth aspect of the right to know, which she calls the "parental disclosure" aspect, which "relates to the right to know the *truth* about the circumstances of one's conception" (668).

want to know is *who* their donor is for reasons that will then answer the question "Who am I?"[19]

This is why I do not argue that intended parents should put their child in a position to acquire relationship genetic knowledge. And it is also why I set aside purely medical or health-related rationales for why intended parents should use an open donor.[20] Appeals to the value of these other kinds of genetic knowledge simply don't reflect the experiences of most donor-conceived people, either by not going far enough (medical genetic knowledge) or going too far (relationship genetic knowledge).

So my focus throughout is on progenitor genetic knowledge where, once again, that denotes knowledge of who their genetic parents are. This might strike some as a limited form of genetic knowledge, leaving out what we might call *ancestral* genetic knowledge, i.e. knowledge of one's genetic lineage going back generations. My focus on progenitor genetic knowledge does not include whatever interest in ancestral genetic knowledge people might have.

There are two reasons for this. First, I think the primary locus of interest for donor-conceived people is knowing who their donor is (even though such knowledge may be a means to acquiring ancestral genetic knowledge). The second reason I focus on progenitor genetic knowledge is that I think there is a strong case for taking seriously a donor-conceived person's interest in acquiring such knowledge. This is because the interest is rationally grounded. I argue in chapters 4 and 5 that it is responsive to something genuinely valuable and not merely a function of living in a bionormative society, i.e. a society that highly valorizes—and often misunderstands—the nature of genetic ties. I am less convinced that the same is true, generally speaking, of people's interest in ancestral genetic knowledge. I will not try to defend that claim here. And, indeed, some of what I say in defense of the interest in acquiring progenitor genetic knowledge can be applied, wholly or in part, in defense of an interest in ancestral genetic knowledge. But I will not make that case, focusing instead on progenitor genetic knowledge.

From here on, I am just going to refer to progenitor genetic knowledge as "genetic knowledge." I grant that shortening it in this way could be misleading, since talk of "genetic knowledge" naturally brings to mind *medical* genetic knowledge. But I'm sticking with the term "genetic knowledge" for

---

[19] Just what counts as an answer to that question and why having progenitor genetic knowledge can help answer it is the topic of chapter 4.

[20] I say more about why I'm setting aside the appeal to medical reasons below (p. 15).

what I'm interested in. The alternatives are either too clunky or no less ambiguous.[21] So, I will use "genetic knowledge" to mean "knowledge of who your genetic progenitors are." Don't forget!

2.3. Anonymous, known, and open donors

Anonymous donors wish to remain unknown—at least at the time of donation—to any of their resulting genetic children.[22] As a result, they donate on the condition that their identities and identifying-information will not be shared with any resulting children without their consent. Here is how NW Cryobank explains things in their FAQ for sperm donors:

> After becoming a qualified sperm donor, you will be issued a donor number and you will only be identified by this number to anyone outside of the donor department. When you retire from the program, it is important that you do not forget your sperm donor number in case you should have questions or any other reason to contact us in the future.
>
> We are obligated by mutual agreements to maintain the anonymity and privacy of all parties, including the donor, recipient, and all offspring resulting from anonymous donor insemination. However, if given mutual consent by the sperm donor and adult offspring, we will attempt to facilitate anonymous contact.[23]

Even if a donor is anonymous, a lot of information is often made available for intended parents—or indeed anyone—to peruse online. This information may include childhood photos, basic facts about appearance (height, eye color, hair color and texture), ethnicity, educational attainment (including areas of study), and a donor "essay" where they respond to prompts like

---

[21] "Biological knowledge," for example, is no less clear. In fact, it is less clear since the genetic relationship is not the only biological relationship present in procreation. A child born of a gestational surrogate might want to know who the surrogate was. This is a kind of biological knowledge. Alternatively, a child who results from an embryo with donated mitochondria might want to know who donated the mitochondria. This is also a kind of biological knowledge. I say a little below about what, if anything, my views about gamete donation mean for these other forms of non-traditional family-making (pp. 25–28).

[22] My description of anonymous donation, open donation, and known donation in the following pages captures the overwhelming majority of gamete donation.

[23] NW Cryobank, "Frequently Asked Questions about Using Donor Sperm," accessed May 19, 2020, https://www.nwcryobank.com/donor-sperm-faqs/.

"Why do you want to be a donor?" and "What is your philosophy of life?"[24] You might also be able to see the Staff Impression of the donor's personality and appearance (e.g. "Lips: Medium fullness to upper lip, full lower lip"). Once someone has selected a donor, even more information might become available. But if the donor is anonymous, no *identifying* information is made available.

It is important to note that "anonymous donor" is a normative category: someone is an anonymous donor in virtue of an understanding with the clinic that their identity *ought* to remain a secret. This means that even if a donor's identity is discovered, he is still an anonymous donor inasmuch as he donated with the understanding that his identity would not be made available to the resulting child or be easily discoverable.[25]

Known donors are known to the intended parents and vice versa from the beginning of the donation process. This is usually because they are a close friend or relative (a brother or a sister, for example) of the intended parents.[26] The child that results from a known donor's gametes usually knows who the donor is and that that person is their donor from a young age.

Open donors typically donate to clinics, which sell the donor's gametes to intended parents, with no input from the donor. Open donors do not know who the intended parents are and vice versa. What makes these donors *open* is that they agree to have their identities revealed to any child that results from their gametes at the child's request when they turn 18 (or before if there is mutual agreement on the matter).[27]

---

[24] Donor 254Z: "As Rocky Balboa says, 'It's not about how hard you hit. It's about how hard you can get hit and keep moving forward, that's how winning is done.'" "Donor Profile," NW Cryobank, accessed January 12, 2021, https://www.nwcryobank.com/donor/.

[25] This last caveat might make some wonder whether there really is such a thing as an anonymous donor in this age of cheap genetic kits and the internet. Perhaps we have reached the end of anonymity when it comes to gamete donation. I discuss this below (p. 12).

[26] Having said that, there has been a considerable rise in the number of people using known donors that are known to them only through the process of trying to find a donor without the aid of clinics altogether. On the rise of donors who are "going direct to customers," see Nellie Bowles, "The Sperm Kings Have a Problem: Too Much Demand," *New York Times*, January 8, 2021, https://www.nytimes.com/2021/01/08/business/sperm-donors-facebook-groups.html.

[27] These kinds of donors are sometimes called "identity-release" donors, although some clinics make a distinction between identity-release donors, who are willing to have their identity released, and open donors who have "agreed to a minimum of one communication with any offspring once he or she turns 18." California Cryobank, "Donor Types," accessed January 12, 2021, https://www.cryobank.com/how-it-works/donor-types/.

3. The central question and the end of anonymity

With these explanations of keys terms in hand, we can make my central claim sharper: intended parents should use an open donor because doing so puts their child in a good position to satisfy the child's likely future interest in progenitor genetic knowledge. But for reasons I've just explained, I'll be sticking with the simpler formulation, which drops "progenitor", throughout: *parents should use an open donor because doing so puts their resulting child in a good position to satisfy the child's likely future interest in having genetic knowledge.*[28]

Some might wonder if, given various advances in genetic testing, anonymous donation is more or less a thing of the past. Remember that "anonymous donor" is a normative category. It picks out donors that reasonably expect their identities to remain unknown to their genetic offspring. But in this age of cheap genetic kits and the internet, can anyone reasonably expect that? Newspapers are rife with articles and advice columns about people who have used a commercially available genetic testing kit and discovered their genetic origins are not at all what they thought they were.[29] The databases of genetic information being compiled by companies such as 23andMe are getting to the point where, "60% of the searches for individuals of European descent will result in a third-cousin or close match, which theoretically allows their identification using demographic identifiers." In the "near future" these kinds of searches "could implicate nearly any U.S. individual of European descent."[30] So, we may be approaching the point where no one can reasonably expect their identity to remain secret and so no one is an anonymous donor.[31]

That might lead some people to think that there's just no point in thinking about the ethics of anonymous versus open donation. But that's not true for

---

[28] This thesis makes a claim about using an *open* donor, not a known donor. That might seem strange since using a known donor puts a child in an even better position to acquire genetic knowledge. I explain why my thesis is about open donors below and then again in chapter 8, (pp. 25–28).

[29] See, for example, Amy Dickinson, "Perspective: Ask Amy: DNA Testing Reveals Shocking Results," *Washington Post*, February 13, 2018, https://www.washingtonpost.com/lifestyle/style/ask-amy-dna-testing-reveals-shocking-results/2018/02/13/54097586-076a-11e8-b48c-b07fea957bd5_story.html; Jacqueline Mroz, "A Mother Learns the Identity of Her Child's Grandmother: A Sperm Bank Threatens to Sue," *New York Times*, February 16, 2019, https://www.nytimes.com/2019/02/16/health/sperm-donation-dna-testing.html; Dani Shapiro, *Inheritance: A Memoir of Genealogy, Paternity, and Love* (New York: Anchor, 2020).

[30] Yaniv Erlich et al., "Identity Inference of Genomic Data Using Long-Range Familial Searches," *Science* 362, no. 6415 (November 9, 2018): 690–94.

[31] Susan Dominus, "Sperm Donors Can't Stay Secret Anymore: Here's What That Means," *New York Times*, June 26, 2019, https://www.nytimes.com/2019/06/26/magazine/sperm-donor-questions.html.

at least the following three reasons. First, even if anonymity could soon be a thing of the past, we're not there yet. There are, then, pressing questions to ask about people who are currently planning to conceive with donated gametes and whose children might be part of a cohort that cannot, as a matter of fact, be confident that they will be able to identity their donor.

Second, even if anonymity becomes a thing of the past, there is a moral difference between parents actively putting their child in a position to acquire genetic knowledge (from someone who is willing to be identified) versus leaving it to the child to track down the information (from a donor who would rather have remained anonymous). If there are good reasons for a donor-conceived person to have access to genetic knowledge, then leaving it to them to track it down (from someone who didn't volunteer to be identified) when their parents could have easily made it available puts the burden on the wrong person.

But are there good reasons for a donor-conceived person to have access to genetic knowledge? This question brings us to the third and most important reason the end of anonymity doesn't render my project irrelevant: pointing out that anonymity is on the way out doesn't shed any *moral* light. That is, it doesn't tell us whether the infeasibility of anonymous donation should be welcomed or lamented. If it should be lamented, then we should consider whether there are policies that could protect or strengthen anonymity (where anonymous donation is still allowed). And perhaps the places where anonymous donation is not permitted should change course! On the other hand, if the end of anonymity is to be welcomed, then we should work toward policies that put the burden of making genetic knowledge available on intended parents and not on their children.

But asking whether we should welcome or lament the end of anonymity matters apart from possible practical ramifications. This is because the question demands that we scrutinize some of our most basic commitments about the nature of families and the ties that bind. As I said earlier, looking closely at the ethics of using an anonymous donor versus an open donor promises to shed light on issues that matter to us all.

4. Framing the issue

Not all intended parents can choose whether to use an anonymous or open donor. As we've already seen, some countries don't permit anonymous donation while others—such as France—require it.[32] But just as the end of anonymity doesn't by itself shed any moral light, neither does the fact that some intended parents can't make a choice about which kind of donor to use. For the questions we should ask are: What options should they have? What should systems of gamete donation and conception look like?

To answer that question, we need to think through the ethics of donor conception quite apart from any particular regulatory system. Once again, we need to know what values are at stake in the choice of using an anonymous or open donor, and whether that choice is actually available to a particular intended parent or not. So when I ask (and answer) the *central question* I am abstracting away from legal and regulatory frameworks that, in fact, limit people's options. Instead, I am wondering about the choice people should make, assuming they have a choice.

Another way of putting this point is that when I ask the *central question*, I am largely setting aside what I call *extrinsic considerations,* by which I mean, simply, considerations generated by features of particular legal or regulatory frameworks for gamete donation. These features might well highly constrain the choices available to intended parents who live under particular frameworks. In taking up the *central question* I focus only on what I call "intrinsic considerations." When I talk about "intrinsic considerations," all I mean is reasons for or against using an open donor that are *not* the result of a particular regulatory framework for donor conception. They are, rather, reasons related to the practice of donor conception that apply no matter what the regulatory framework is.

Crucially, although I am abstracting away from the details of any particular regulatory framework, my project is firmly grounded in what procreation, parenting, and being a donor-conceived person are like for human beings in our world. I am not interested in the ethics of donor conception for any possible creature (that needs gametes for procreation) or in circumstances that are radically different from those in our world. The *central question* would no doubt be answered differently if we could fend for ourselves minutes after being born or if our phenotypes had almost nothing to do with genetics or if we tended not to form any special emotional attachment with the people who raise us. So I'll say it again (because it's important): talk of "intrinsic

---

[32] Although people can, and routinely do, travel to nearby countries where they can make the choice they want to. For discussion of this practice in the UK, see Ilke Turkmendag, "When Sperm Cannot Travel: Experiences of UK Would-Be Parents Seeking Treatment Abroad," *European Law and New Health Technologies*, 2013, pp. 362–380.

considerations" is *not* meant to suggest that we should try to think about the ethics of donor conception in any possible world. Instead, it is meant to pick out features of donor conception that will be present in any plausible system for donor conception in our world, for creatures like us.

5. Setting aside the Medical Reasons view

I've already told you my answer to the *central question*: parents should use an open donor because doing so puts their resulting child in a good position to satisfy the child's likely future interest in having genetic knowledge. One obvious source of that likely future interest is that having genetic knowledge can be critically important for medical reasons.

The Medical Reasons view (as I'll call it) is certainly plausible, as the following example makes clear:

> In 2009, a single mother of donor-conceived twins took legal action to force the New England Cryogenic Center to reveal the identity and medical records of her donor after her daughters were diagnosed with a growth disorder and other "health crises" that—according to her—they inherited from the donor. She explained that doctors struggled to correctly diagnose their condition, which would have been easier to diagnose if she had access to the donor's medical family history.[33]

Things can also work the other way around. A donor-conceived person might mistakenly believe he is genetically prone to get a condition because his non-genetic social parent has it. Suppose a donor-conceived person's father and grandfather developed early onset dementia. And suppose he believes that they are all genetically related. He would then reasonably believe that he is at serious risk of early onset dementia. Needless to say, this would cause considerable stress.[34]

So case closed. The Medical Reasons view explains why intended parents should not use an anonymous donor. But concluding that intended parents

---

[33] Ravitsky, "Knowing Where You Come From," 671. The case she mentions was originally reported in the *Boston Herald*, but the stories don't appear to be online anymore.

[34] A story like this with respect to the BRCA gene appears in Diane Ehrensaft, *Mommies, Daddies, Donors, Surrogates: Answering Tough Questions and Building Strong Families* (New York: Guilford Press, 2005), 157.

should not use an anonymous donor simply on the basis of the Medical Reasons view is not satisfying for at least two reasons. First, it is hardly clear that the medical challenges that can arise with anonymous donation require that donor-conceived people know the *identity* of their donor. This is especially clear in the dementia case: the stress of worrying that one might have inherited a propensity for dementia would be alleviated by simply knowing that one is not genetically related to one's father.[35]

Admittedly, cases of the first kind—where the medical issue was inherited from the donor—are different. But even here, it's not clear that the donor-conceived person needs to know the identity of the donor rather than facts about the donor's genome and medical history. It could be true that, as a matter of fact, the most effective way to learn facts of this sort is to know who the donor is. But we might imagine a regime of gamete donation where detailed genomic and medical information is kept on hand, updated over the years, and made available to donor-conceived people.[36] Apart from that possibility, we are perhaps not so far from being able to extract whatever important medical information we need directly from the genomic profile of the patient himself, rendering knowing one's family history unimportant.[37] What all this suggests is that the move from "This person is donor-conceived" to "There are decisive medical reasons for them to know the identity of their donor" is not as airtight as it seems.

But even if it were airtight—even if, that is, there were decisive medical reasons for ensuring that donor-conceived people know the identity of their donors—there is a second reason why we should not rest content with the Medical Reasons view: it short-circuits exploration of whether there are other, perhaps more significant, reasons for intended parents to use an open donor. The Medical Reasons view bypasses altogether questions about the value of genetic knowledge that have nothing to do with medical well-being. These are questions about the place of genetic knowledge in understanding oneself and one's place in the world. The Medical Reasons view might return the *verdict* many donor-conceived people want, but fails to acknowledge the *reasons* for the verdict that at least some donor-conceived people would appeal to:

---

[35] Knowing this would raise all kinds of other questions (like: "Who *is* my genetic father?"). These kinds of questions are central to my argument. The important point here is that such questions move us beyond the Medical Reasons view.

[36] Or their parents, if needed, when the donor-conceived person is a child.

[37] Inmaculada De Melo-Martín, "The Ethics of Anonymous Gamete Donation: Is There a Right to Know One's Genetic Origins?," *Hastings Center Report* 44, no. 2 (2014): 31.

I got the impression that "society" didn't feel I have a right to anything more than a medical history. People don't acknowledge a need/right to know traits, history, or even realize that their sense of identity might be tied up with their family history, or family stories, or remembrances about a person.[38]

The fact that some donor-conceived people attribute significance to genetic knowledge that goes beyond any medical significance it might have doesn't mean that they are right to do so. So my point here is not that we should just endorse the idea that genetic knowledge is significant for reasons that go beyond whatever medical significance it might have. Rather, my point is that there are deep and difficult questions to grapple with, questions that won't be asked if we stop at the idea that there are decisive medical reasons for using an open donor. We can reformulate the *central question* to capture this line of thought: Should intended parents use an open donor even if there were no medical reasons for doing so?

6. Setting aside an appeal to rights

You might think that the *central question* is easily answered for the following reason: people have a *right* to know who their genetic progenitors are. The appeal to the "right to know" usually takes one of two forms. According to the first, the right to know is *basic* in the sense that it is not derivative of some other right. Conceiving with anonymously donated gametes, on this view, effectively violates this right.[39] According to the second view, the right to know is derivative of a more general autonomy right that people have to shape their identity as they see fit, including by appeal to facts about their genetic

---

[38] Amanda J. Turner and Adrian Coyle, "What Does It Mean to Be a Donor Offspring? The Identity Experiences of Adults Conceived by Donor Insemination and the Implications for Counselling and Therapy," *Human Reproduction* 15, no. 9 (2000): 2047.

[39] Austria's Medically Assisted Procreation Act 1992 interpreted Article 7 of the United Nations Conventions on the Rights of the Child as articulating such a right. Article 7 reads, "The child shall be registered immediately after birth and shall have the right from birth to a name, the right to acquire a nationality and, as far as possible, *the right to know and be cared for by his or her parents*" (emphasis added). As Lucy Frith points out, this hardly provides unambiguous support for the "right to know." The Austrian legislation seemed to interpolate a particular, and contentious, understanding of what "parent" means in the article above. Lucy Frith, "Gamete Donation and Anonymity: The Ethical and Legal Debate," *Human Reproduction* 16, no. 5 (2001): 818–24. Frith also discusses how the Basic Rights view has been appealed to in the formulation of legislation in Australia and Switzerland. Lucy Frith, "Beneath the Rhetoric: The Role of Rights in the Practice of Non-Anonymous Gamete Donation," *Bioethics* 15, nos. 5–6 (2001): 820–21.

progenitors. Conceiving a person *via* anonymous donation effectively closes the door to that person constructing her identity in this way.[40]

Beyond what I say here, I neither take up nor take on these rights-based answers to the *central question*. This isn't because I deny that donor-conceived people have a right to know.[41] Rather, it is because I see rights-based views as (at best) the start, and not the end, of arguments about the ethics of conceiving with anonymously donated gametes. Perhaps it is right to say, "Parents should use an open donor because their child is entitled to genetic knowledge. They have a right to know." But we should also ask: *Why* is the child entitled to genetic knowledge? And to answer that question we need to know what goods, interests, and values are at stake.[42] The Nuffield Council on Bioethics puts this point very well in their report *Donor Conception: Ethical Aspects of Information Sharing*:

> Starting from the language of rights . . . is effectively to start with conclusions: the conclusion that particular interests are of sufficient importance to impose duties on others to ensure that the right-holder is able to enjoy the interest in question. Using the language of interests, on the other hand, enables us first to unpack what we know about the nature of those interests, and then go on to consider at a second stage the extent to which others might be held to bear responsibilities in connection with the promotion or protection of those interests.[43]

[40] Though Feinberg is not concerned with this particular issue, his argument could easily be used to support this view. Joel Feinberg, "The Child's Right to an Open Future," in *Justice, Politics, and the Family* (New York: Routledge, 2015), 145–60. The view is argued for explicitly in Vardit Ravitsky, "Autonomous Choice and the Right to Know One's Genetic Origins," *Hastings Center Report* 44, no. 2 (2014): 36–37. Olivia Pratten is a Canadian woman who, at age 28, sued the province of British Columbia in 2010 for access to records concerning her donor (after unsuccessfully trying to get access to the records herself for almost 10 years). She articulates her reasoning for wanting the information in a way that aligns with the Derivative Right view: "We each choose to construct our identities in different ways. Some people embrace identity through their families and through their biological ties. For some, identity is constructed solely from a cultural group affiliation or from other non-blood relationships. [. . .] I aim to gain control of how I choose to construct my identity." See Pratten's contribution in Juliet Ruth Guichon, Ian Mitchell, and Michelle Giroux, eds., *The Right to Know One's Origins: Assisted Human Reproduction and the Best Interests of Children* (Brussels: ASP, 2012), 51. Pratten won her initial case, but the decision was overturned by the British Columbia Court of Appeals. In 2013, the Canadian Supreme Court refused to take up the case.

[41] I confess that I'm not sure what I think on this matter. But I don't feel much pressure to resolve my uncertainty since, for reasons I'm about to explain, I think the central question can be answered without an appeal to rights at all.

[42] For a compelling account of what grounds children's rights and the nature of the different goods at play, see Samantha Brennan, "The Goods of Childhood, Children's Rights, and the Role of Parents as Advocates and Interpreters," in *Family-Making: Contemporary Ethical Challenges*, ed. F. Baylis and C. McLeod (New York, n.d.), 29–48.

[43] Nuffield Council on Bioethics, *Donor Conception: Ethical Aspects of Information Sharing* (London: Nuffield Council on Bioethics, 2013), 86.

This point applies to both basic and derivative versions of the rights-based approach. If the right to know is basic (in the sense that it is not derived from some other, more fundamental right), then we need to know why genetic knowledge is so important that there is a basic right to it.

A slightly more complicated version of this point applies to the view that the right to know is derived from the autonomy right to determine one's identity as one sees fit. On this picture, a huge part of the value undergirding the right to know is the value of autonomy or self-determination.[44] Naturally, one might have all kinds of questions about the nature and value of autonomy. But the point that interests me here is that even if we grant that autonomy is hugely valuable *and* that identity determination is a central part of being autonomous, we still need an account of why genetic knowledge must be made available in the pool of materials from which to construct one's identity.[45] Consider the myriad of utterly trivial facts about yourself, both past and present, that pass by entirely unnoticed and without playing any role whatsoever in your self-understanding. There is no right to know what color socks the mailman was wearing on the day you were conceived or how much gas was in the family car when you turned 3. More generally, there is no expectation that a person has access to every bit of information about themselves in order to be able to determine their identity in accordance with the dictates of autonomy. Parents don't do anything wrong by failing to record, notice, care about, pay attention to, or share with their child *all kinds* of information about their child, let alone the circumstances of the child's conception.

What matters for identity determination is that someone has access to information about themselves that *really matters*, the *important stuff*. And the implicit idea behind the claim that people have a right to genetic knowledge (as part of a larger autonomy right) is that it really matters. Having access to genetic knowledge is not on a par with knowing what color socks the mailman was wearing the day you were conceived. It is not trivial.

Whether some version of that claim is right is the topic of chapters 3 through 5. Taken together they aim to show that a donor-conceived person's interest in genetic knowledge is weighty indeed. So, even though I do not pursue a rights-based argument, nothing I say is at odds with that conclusion. Indeed, my argument could, perhaps, be taken to provide the underlying rationale for a rights-based view.[46]

---

[44] Ravitsky, "Autonomous Choice and the Right to Know One's Genetic Origins."

[45] Just what it means to "determine" or "construct" one's identity is discussed in detail in chapter 4.

[46] Thank you to Samantha Brennan for helpful discussion on how my view might go with a rights-based account.

7. Outline of the book

Here's my argument in a nutshell: the fact that a donor-conceived person is likely to be very interested in acquiring genetic knowledge gives intended parents a weighty reason to use an open donor. Parents ought to promote their children's well-being by helping satisfy their child's worthwhile significant interests, and a donor-conceived person's interest in genetic knowledge is one such interest. Moreover, the weighty reason to use an open donor usually provides a *decisive* reason to use an open donor. So, more intended parents should use an open donor. I call this the Significant Interest view.

The Significant Interest view turns on the empirical claim that many donor-conceived people have a weighty interest in genetic knowledge. As we will see, this interest is not merely a proxy or evidence for some other consideration in favor of using an open donor. Instead, it is itself a crucial part of the story for why intended parents should use an open donor. If it turned out that most donor-conceived people were basically uninterested in who their genetic parents are—seeing it, perhaps, as no more interesting than the color of the mailman's socks on the day they were conceived—then my argument would fail.

In this respect, my view is firmly grounded in the social science about new family forms and, more specifically, families constituted by means of donor conception.[47] One thing I try to do throughout the book is to stay true to the voices of donor-conceived people, simultaneously taking seriously that the majority are interested in obtaining genetic knowledge, while also acknowledging that a significant portion are not.[48] A consequence of building my argument around what donor-conceived people are, for the most part, actually interested in is that my view has a kind of contingency to it that is often absent (or at least purportedly absent) from philosophical arguments. If facts about people's psychology were very different or were to change—absent coercion or undue influence—then my conclusion would probably be very different. The philosophical purists in the crowd might see this aspect of my work as a bug. I prefer to see it as a feature.

---

[47] I discuss the social science in various places throughout the book, but Susan Golombok's *Modern Families* has been my go-to resource on this front. I highly recommend it to anyone interested in a quick and highly readable overview of the relevant social science. Susan Golombok, *Modern Families: Parents and Children in New Family Forms* (Cambridge: Cambridge University Press, 2015).

[48] I discuss these empirical claims in chapter 3. The fact that it is not uncommon to find donor-conceived people who have no real interest in obtaining genetic knowledge plays a crucial role in my defense of the Significant Interest view.

In chapter 2, I offer a novel argument for the claim that (generally) parents who conceive a child with donated gametes should disclose to their child that she is donor-conceived whether or not they plan to use an anonymous donor. The argument for using an open donor begins in chapter 3, where I present the Significant Interest view. I argue that because a donor-conceived child is very likely to develop a worthwhile significant interest in acquiring genetic knowledge, parents have a weighty reason to avoid using an anonymous donor. This reason is grounded in parents' obligation to help their children satisfy their worthwhile significant interests.

It might look as though the Significant Interest view is fatally vulnerable to one of two very different objections. First, it appears that the view is parasitic on the claim that genetic knowledge *really matters*, that it has value apart from a person's subjective interest in it. After all, the Significant Interest view claims that a person's significant interest in genetic knowledge is *worthwhile*. But then, the objection goes, the Significant Interest view is a kind of sideshow: if a person's interest in genetic knowledge is worthwhile, then the case for using an open donor should go directly through the claim that having genetic knowledge is valuable and *not* through what appears to be a mere symptom of its value, namely that many people are interested in having it.

The Sideshow objection is motivated by the thought that the Significant Interest view undersells the extent to which genetic knowledge really matters. The second objection is motivated by the thought that the Significant Interest view *oversells* that idea. According to the Bionormativity objection, the idea that an interest in genetic knowledge is worthwhile is suspect:[49] people's interest in genetic knowledge is plausibly trivial or, worse, morally problematic in virtue of evincing a kind of bionormative prejudice, i.e. a set of attitudes, beliefs, and practices that unjustifiably valorizes genetic ties and the "bionormative family."[50] If that's right, then the idea that parents are obligated to help their children satisfy an interest in acquiring genetic knowledge is highly suspect.

Considered in tandem, the objections suggest that the Significant Interest view is unstable: it either collapses into the view that having genetic knowledge really matters or it dissolves altogether. I address the Sideshow and

---

[49] Bearing in mind that we are setting aside the Medical Reasons view.

[50] Charlotte Witt, "Family, Self and Society: A Critique of the Bionormative Conception of the Family," in *Family-Making: Contemporary Ethical Challenges*, ed. Carolyn MacLeod Francois Baylis (New York: Oxford University Press, 2014). Motivating this claim, which I think presents a serious challenge to my view, is one of the tasks of chapter 5.

Bionormativity objections in chapters 4 and 5. In chapter 4, I argue that genetic knowledge has optional prudential value as part of the necessary task
of identity determination. The simple idea at the heart of that chapter is
this: genetic knowledge can, but need not, play a central role in efforts to
answer the question "Who am I?" This question often comes up in donor-
conceived people's accounts of why they want genetic knowledge. Among
other things, I offer an analysis of what exactly the question is asking and
how having genetic knowledge can and cannot contribute to answering it.
The upshot of this chapter is that the case for using an open donor cannot
appeal directly to the value of genetic knowledge, but must appeal instead to
the fact that donor-conceived people generally *want* genetic knowledge. The
appeal to donor-conceived people's actual interest in genetic knowledge is
not a sideshow.

In chapter 5, I consider whether people's interest in acquiring genetic
knowledge is morally problematic. This might, on the face of it, sound like an
implausible view. Properly understood, however, the claim has a lot of force.
One central goal of this chapter is to show why that is. But the second central
goal is to show that the sense in which it is plausible does not threaten the
Significant Interest view.

Having defended the Significant Interest view from the sideshow and
bionormativity objections, I argue in chapter 6 that the weighty reason
parents have to use an open donor is usually decisive. In other words, I show
that when we consider the reasons that, in general, intended parents might
have to use an anonymous donor alongside the weighty reason to use an
open donor, the latter (usually) wins out. The conclusion is that, in general,
intended parents should use an open donor.

In chapter 7 I turn to the role and responsibility of the donor. I argue that
while gamete donation is the kind of activity that triggers parental responsibilities, donors never actually incur parental responsibilities. Instead, they
incur intended parental responsibilities, which in the normal course of things
are transferred to intended parents before there is ever a child to be parentally responsible *to*. The key thought here is that the gap between the time of
donation and the time a child is actually conceived allows for the transfer of
who will be parentally responsible in the first place. So, donors are typically
never parentally responsible for the children that result from their gametes.
Even so, I argue, the Significant Interest view dictates that prospective donors
should be open donors. If parents ought to use an open donor, then donors
ought to choose to be open donors lest they implicate themselves in a morally

problematic practice. The upshot is that prospective donors must be willing to be known and, realistically, contacted by their genetic offspring.

In the final chapter of the book, I turn to questions of policy and, in particular, whether the state should legally prohibit anonymous donation. My answer, perhaps surprisingly given my central thesis, is that it should not. The longer answer is that efforts to outlaw anonymous gamete donation must be accompanied, if not preceded by, efforts to undo bionormative prejudice. As I see it, intended parents should not choose an anonymous donor. But there are *lots* of things parents should not do but which they are nonetheless permitted to do. Choosing an anonymous donor is, in my view, one of those things. Using the state's coercive power to prevent parents from making a mistake that is of a kind we generally allow parents to make threatens to further stigmatize family-forms that are already stigmatized.

8. "Would you rather not exist?"

Some readers might think my whole approach really misses the boat because of this point: children conceived with anonymously donated gametes would not exist had their parents chosen an open donor (different donor = different person coming into existence). And this might lead some people to doubt that there are any possible grounds for a donor-conceived person to complain about having been brought into existence without access to genetic knowledge. "Surely," the thought goes, "the lives of donor-conceived people are worth living even if they lack genetic knowledge." And surely they are. "But then," says the critic, "people conceived with anonymously donated gametes have nothing to complain about. They have lives well worth living, which they would not have had if their parents had used an open donor. For in that case, they wouldn't exist at all! So what is there to complain about?"[51]

This line of thought isn't compelling. The fact that a life is worth living is not a sufficient condition for permissibly creating it. A striking illustration of this idea can be found in Kazuo Ishiguro's book *Never Let Me Go* (spoiler alert), where clones are created to ensure a steady supply of organs

---

[51] Philosophers will recognize this as a version of the non-identity problem. The website We Are Donor Conceived has a page devoted to this line of thought. See Jonathan Pollack, "Would You Rather Not Exist?," *We Are Donor Conceived*, accessed January 5th, 2020, https://www.wearedonorconceived. com/personal-stories/would-you-rather-not-exist/

for (non-clone) people who need them.[52] The clones are treated very well and generally lead moderately fulfilling lives . . . until they are called on to give up an organ. And even then, they might continue to live moderately good lives if they don't strictly need the organ they've given up . . . until they are called on again to give more organs. The book is deeply troubling and, at times, un-speakably sad, even though the people who are used for their organs quite clearly have lives worth living. And this is precisely because there are ways of creating people that are at odds with the value of personhood even if the resulting lives are (well) worth living.

The question is whether creating people with anonymously donated gametes is one of those ways. No one, I take it, will think it is quite so bad as creating people to painlessly harvest their organs later in life. But there are those who think that depriving people of genetic knowledge is bad *enough* that it is fundamentally disrespectful to create people using anonymously donated gametes (even if the people's lives are well worth living).[53]

For reasons that will become clear as the book proceeds, I don't believe that creating a child with anonymously donated gametes is fundamentally disrespectful of their personhood. I think people shouldn't do it, but I don't think it's *that* bad. Even so, I think the underlying thought is right: if we have choices about the kind of people we create, we have a weighty reason to create the people whose lives will go best.[54] People who plan to conceive with donated gametes have a choice about whom to create based, in part, on whether they use an anonymous or open donor. If, as I will argue, there are good reasons to think it is better for the resulting child to have access to ge-netic knowledge, then intended parents have a weighty reason to use an open donor. And this is true even if the child who would result from anonymously donated gametes would have had a life well worth living. So, conceiving a person with anonymously donated gametes cannot be justified *simply* on the

---

[52] Ishiguro, Kazuo. *Never Let Me Go*. 2010.

[53] This line of thought is developed by David Velleman, who casts doubt on the concept of a "life worth living," preferring instead to think in terms of lives worth continuing versus lives worth cre-ating. I say more about this aspect of Velleman's view in chapter 3. J. David Velleman, "III. Love and Nonexistence," *Philosophy & Public Affairs* 36, no. 3 (2008): 266–88.

[54] This is a simplified version of what Kahane and Savulescu call the *Principle of Procreative Beneficence*:

> If couples (or single reproducers) have decided to have a child and selection is possible, then they have a significant moral reason to select the child, of the possible children they could have, whose life can be expected, in light of the relevant available information, to go best or at least not worse than any of the others.

Julian Savulescu and Guy Kahane, "The Moral Obligation to Create Children with the Best Chance of the Best Life," *Bioethics* 23, no. 5 (2009): 274.

grounds that the person's life will be worth living. If intended parents can create a person who, as far as they know, will have a better life than some other person they might create, then they have a weighty reason to create the first person.[55]

9. What about known donors?

As you go through the book, you might wonder whether the arguments I make for using an open donor do not, in fact, establish that intended parents should use a *known* donor. Maybe they do, but I am not confident on this point. My case for using an open donor depends not only on the interest a donor-conceived person is likely to have in genetic knowledge, but also on the comparative unimportance of whatever interests intended parents have in using an anonymous donor. The "comparative" is really important here. In a number of places, I consider the very real considerations that might incline intended parents to want to use an anonymous donor and find them wanting when put alongside the reason for using an open donor.

By contrast, the reasons intended parents might have for preferring an open donor to a known donor are not, in my view, comparatively unimportant when put alongside whatever reasons there are to use known donors. Conceiving with a known donor introduces complications for intended parents—primary among them are *finding* a known donor and then negotiating what role that person should have in the resultant child's life from the get-go. Those complications are not present, at least not with the same acuity, when it comes to using an open donor. So, even though I am confident that my argument shows that, usually, people ought to use an open donor, I'm not at all confident it shows that they ought to use a known donor.

10. Other forms of non-traditional family-making: adoption, surrogacy, and mitochondrial donation

Donor conception is just one kind of non-traditional family-making. Some families are formed through adoption. Others come about through use of a gestational surrogate. And some come about via mitochondrial donation,

---

[55] And, if what I argue in chapter 5 is right, usually a decisive reason.

where a donor's mitochondria replace the mitochondria in the egg that will be used for conception so as to avoid mitochondrial diseases.[56] How does my account of the ethics of donor conception relate to these other forms of family-making?

The short answer is this: my view implies that parents who engage in these other forms of family-making should not use third parties who will remain unknown to the resulting child *if* there is good reason to think that child will develop a significant worthwhile interest in knowing who that third party is. So, for example, if children who are gestated by surrogates tend to develop a significant interest in knowing who gestated them, then intended parents should use gestational surrogates who agree to be known to the resulting child.[57] The same goes for mitochondrial donation.

But whether my account straightforwardly extends to these other kinds of cases depends on how we answer one philosophical question and one empirical question. The philosophical question is this: Does my account of why people's interest in genetic knowledge is worthwhile apply, either entirely or partly, to the interests people might have in knowing who their mitochondrial donor is or who their gestational parent is?[58] As I argue in chapter 4, genetic knowledge can play a central role in answering the question "Who am I?" One of the points I make there is that this question itself can be broken down into a series of what I call *identity questions*: How am I? What am I (like)? Who am I like? These identity questions are not all about the same sense of "identity": some have to do with metaphysical or numerical identity, while others have to do with the *kind* of person one is. The point here is just that it is not immediately clear how the other interests we're now considering—to know, for example, who one's mitochondrial donor is—intersects with the different senses of identity implicated in the identity questions.[59]

---

[56] These are known as "three parent" cases.

[57] One might think that creating children *via* gestational surrogacy is deeply problematic in the first place. See, for example, Anca Gheaus, "Biological Parenthood: Gestational, Not Genetic," *Australasian Journal of Philosophy* 96, no. 2 (April 3, 2018): 225–40. For a different kind of critique, see Debra Satz, "Markets in Women's Reproductive Labor," *Philosophy & Public Affairs* 21, no. 2 (1992): 107–31. I take no stand on the ethics of gestational surrogacy.

[58] Since birth mothers are genetically related to the children, the story I tell in chapter 3 applies straightaway to the interest in knowing one's birth mother. The question in this case is whether my story is the *whole* story. I doubt it is.

[59] For discussion of these issues, see Anthony Wrigley, Stephen Wilkinson, and John B. Appleby, "Mitochondrial Replacement: Ethics and Identity," *Bioethics* 29, no. 9 (2015): 631–38. See also Ilke Turkmendag, "It Is Just a 'Battery': 'Right' to Know in Mitochondrial Replacement," *Science, Technology, & Human Values* 43, no. 1 (January 1, 2018): 56–85.

The empirical question is this: Are children who are created by some forms of non-traditional family-making more likely to want to know the identity of the "third party" (the birth mother, the gestational surrogate, the gamete donor, the mitochondrial donor) than others? It is very common for (gamete) donor-conceived children to want to know who their donor is. Will the same be true for children conceived with donated mitochondria, for example? If it turns out that they are largely indifferent to know who their mitochondrial donor is, then my case for using an open gamete donor just won't apply to mitochondrial donation.

Where does the voluminous sociological (and less voluminous philosophical) work on adoption fit into my view? I occasionally appeal to some of it, but for the most part I set it aside for two related reasons. First, even though it is true that sociological investigation of families with donor-conceived children—and in particular the thoughts and feelings of donor-conceived children themselves—is in its relative infancy compared to the sociology of adoption, there is nonetheless a decent amount of research about donor-conceived children and their families.[60]

Second, and more significantly, the practice of adoption comes with various confounding factors that make it less than ideal as a site for thinking about the value of genetic knowledge. First, adopted children are gestated by their genetic mothers, and the gestational relationship is plausibly significant for both (gestational) mother and child. Second, adopted children have been relinquished, or "given up," by someone—namely the birth mother—with whom the child has plausibly established a significant relationship (i.e. at least the relationship of gestation, but oftentimes something much beyond that if the child was put up for adoption after being cared for by its birth mother or someone else for months or years).[61] Third, and relatedly, adoption more or less always happen in the context of difficult circumstances for the birth mother, circumstances that explain why the resulting child was "given

---

[60] Having said that, a lot of the research in this area suffers from small sample sizes and real concerns about selection bias. I say a little more about this in chapter 3.

[61] According to the Adoption Network, "About 135,000 children are adopted in the United States each year. Of non-stepparent adoptions, about 59% are from the child welfare (or foster) system, 26% are from other countries, and 15% are voluntarily relinquished American babies." As most adoptions happen through the foster care system, "[t]he average child waits for an adoptive family for more than three years. 11 percent spend 5 years or more waiting for a family (43,083 children). The average age of children waiting for an adoptive family is 8." Sixty-two percent of children adopted in a private adoption "were placed with their adoptive families within a month of birth." Adoption Network, "US Adoption Statistics," accessed August 3, 2020, https://adoptionnetwork.com/adoption-statistics.

up."[62] In some cases, the child was not "wanted" in the first place. But in many cases, the child very much *was* wanted, and loved, by the birth mother, but the child was placed in foster care for their own good.[63]

Taken together, these considerations make adoption fraught. The adopted child (who knows they are adopted) must contend—as part of their story about themselves—with having been gestated by their genetic mother, but nonetheless relinquished either because they were, in some sense, not wanted in the first place or in spite of the fact that they were. I don't mean to suggest that all adopted children care about the circumstances of their adoption, that one can't "contend" with these features by simply not caring. But certainly many adopted people do care. This is not to say adopted people do not care about the genetic link as such. My point is just that when it comes to adoption, the issue of genetic relatedness is bound up with so many other things.

This is typically not true when it comes to donor conception. The absent genetic parent is not the gestational parent; the child was wanted (indeed intentionally created) from the get-go; the child is not "given up" by anyone with whom they have a significant relationship via gestation or social ties; and finally, the circumstances of the child coming into the world or being separated from a genetic parent are not "difficult." Indeed, on the usual way of thinking about donor conception, the link between the absent genetic parent(s) and the resulting child is *only* genetic. By "only" here I don't mean to suggest insignificance (e.g. "It's only a paper moon"). That would be to entirely prejudge one of the central issues in the book. Rather, the point is that the genetic link is the *sole* link. There are not confounding features built into the very structure of donor conception that make it difficult to get the genetic link in view. On the contrary: when it comes to donor conception, there isn't really anything else to look at.

---

[62] I don't mean to suggest that adoption, or families constituted by adoption, are "second best." Indeed, I do not think they are. But it is undeniable that in almost all cases of actual adoption, the fact of adoption is evidence for the genetic/gestational mother being in a difficult situation: the fact of adoption is, from her point of view at least, not ideal (even if it is for the best). It is a mistake, however, to infer from the fact that it is not ideal for the genetic/gestational mother that it is therefore not ideal, or not as things should go, for the child.

[63] Although oftentimes the choice (if it is fair to call it that at all) was absurdly constrained. For what this looked like for a certain generation of mothers who gave up their children for adoption, see Ann Fessler, *The Girls Who Went Away: The Hidden History of Women Who Surrendered Children for Adoption in the Decades before Roe v. Wade* (New York: Penguin, 2007).

11. "Do I have to read the whole book?"

While this book argues for a central thesis, it is largely modular. If you are mostly interested in the grounds of parental responsibility and whether donors are parentally responsible you can read chapter 7 on its own. If you are largely interested in the value of genetic knowledge, you can just read chapter 4 (although I would suggest reading chapter 5 as well). If you're interested largely in the ethics of disclosure, just read chapter 2 and stop there. While each chapter is framed in terms of the overall argument of the book, the arguments within each chapter are largely self-standing. But go on, read the whole thing![64]

---

[64] Follow Weinberg's advice: "From cover to cover. At least twice. And then a third time with musical and alcoholic accompaniment." Okay, that was about *her* book, but I'm sure she thinks it about mine too. Weinberg, *The Risk of a Lifetime*, 12.

2

Keeping Secrets

For the child's sake particularly I prefer that absolutely nobody but the parents themselves should know of the insemination therapy. My last advice to the parents is that under no circumstances should they, or need they, ever tell the child about the method of conception—in fact they should forget about it themselves.

—Philip Bloom, *The Eugenics Review*, 1957

What never fails to draw me in . . . are secrets. Secrets within families. Secrets we keep out of shame, or self-protectiveness, or denial. Secrets and their corrosive power. Secrets we keep from one another in the name of love.

—Dani Shapiro, *Inheritance: A Memoir of Genealogy, Paternity, and Love*, 2020

Dani Shapiro was 54 when she compared the results of her commercial ancestry DNA kit to that of the woman she had always thought was her half-sister. The results said otherwise: there was no genetic connection between them. Thus begins the Shapiro's story, recounted in her memoir *Inheritance*, of coming to learn that she is donor-conceived. Shapiro's story is hardly unique. Online resources for donor-conceived people are replete with accounts of people learning late in life—often by accident—that they are donor-conceived.

Many such stories come from people, like Shapiro, who were conceived in the early days of widespread donor conception. The advice back then from the experts ("experts") was to keep the fact that one's child was donor-conceived a complete secret. Non-disclosure was not presented as a moral option but rather something like a moral *requirement*, grounded in claims about the welfare of the child and the privacy of the parents:

Conceiving People. Daniel Groll, Oxford University Press. © Oxford University Press 2021.
DOI: 10.1003/ooo/9780190063054.003.0002

Nondisclosure has traditionally been employed to achieve several goals. It is seen as a way to ensure that the non-genetic parent be perceived as equally connected to the child, to ensure that the child grows as strong a bond with that parent as with the genetic parent, to maintain the appearance of a "normal" family, to avoid distressing the child with the truth of his/her origin, and to allow the nongenetic parent's infertility—a condition that usually carries a negative stigma with it—to remain unknown to other people.[1]

Times have changed. Disclosure is now recommended. The Ethics Committee of the American Society for Reproductive Medicine, for example, says that "[w]hile ultimately the choice of recipient parents, disclosure to offspring of the use of donor gametes in encouraged."[2] Non-disclosure is not an option for some families: lesbian couples and women who choose to raise a child on their own will need to let the child know, at some point, the circumstances of their conception.[3] But heterosexual couples can realistically keep the child's donor conception a secret.

Most still do. According to Susan Golombok:

> In the European Study of Assisted Reproduction Families, not one set of the participating 111 donor insemination parents from Italy, Spain, the Netherlands and the UK has disclosed the donor conception to their children by the time their children were early school age, less than 10 percent of parents had done so by the time their children were in early adolescence, and a follow-up study of the UK sample found that no further children has been told by the time they were 18 years old. [...] Even in Sweden, where legislation giving donor offspring the right to obtain information about the donor's identity came into force in 1985, more than a decade later, only 11 percent of parents were found to have informed their children of their donor conception. Investigations in the USA have produced comparable

---

[1] Glenn McGee, Sarah-Vaughan Brakman, and Andrea D. Gurmankin, "Gamete Donation and Anonymity: Disclosure to Children Conceived with Donor Gametes Should Not Be Optional," *Human Reproduction* 16, no. 10 (2001): 2034.

[2] Medicine, Ethics Committee of the American Society for Reproductive Medicine, "Informing Offspring of Their Conception by Gamete Donation," *Fertility and Sterility* 81, no. 3 (2004): 527.

[3] Although it is true that a single mother could easily lie about those circumstances so as to leave out the fact that her child was donor-conceived. The lesbian couple could too, I suppose, but not so easily.

findings, with rate of disclosure to children reported to range between 14 and 30 percent.[4]

Some parents decide in advance that they will not tell their child they are donor-conceived. Other parents intend to, but struggle to find the supposedly "right time."[5]

The goal of this chapter is to argue that, normally, parents should tell their donor-conceived child that they (the children) are donor-conceived. The "normally" is important. It will be easy to think of cases where keeping *the secret*, as I shall call it, is justified. Perhaps the fate of the world depends on keeping it! The interesting question is whether in general—and not in certain, unusual cases—it is permissible to keep *the secret*. I will argue that it is not.

I start by discussing three standard arguments for disclosure. I reject one of them but think the other two are quite powerful. Even so, I do not think they tell the whole story. As a result, I develop a novel argument for disclosure that turns on the demands of intimacy in the parent-child relationship. As part of this argument, I show that non-disclosure is properly thought of as keeping a secret and that it is deceptive. Finally, I argue that (normally) parents should not keep *the secret* whether or not they intend to use an anonymous donor.

Before we get going, we need to distinguish between two questions we might be asking. First: Should parents keep *the secret* in the first place? Second: Should parents who are keeping *the secret* continue to keep it? My focus is on the first question. This is in keeping with my overall approach to thinking through the ethics of gamete donation: the task is to think about the choices intended parents should make from the beginning (assuming they have choices). The central choice I'm concerned with is whether to choose an anonymous or an open donor. In this chapter, however, I focus on whether to disclose to one's child that they are donor-conceived.

So the central claim of this chapter is that parents should not keep *the secret* in the first place. The situation is decidedly more complex when it comes to parents who face social circumstances that make disclosure a costly

---

[4] Susan Golombok, *Modern Families: Parents and Children in New Family Forms* (Cambridge, UK: Cambridge University Press, 2015), 99.

[5] Ann Lalos, Claes Gottlieb, and Othon Lalos, "Legislated Right for Donor-Insemination Children to Know Their Genetic Origin: A Study of Parental Thinking," *Human Reproduction* 22, no. 6 (2007): 1763.

prospect[6] or parents who are currently keeping *the secret*. The reasons I identity for not keeping *the secret* in the first place certainly apply to both kinds
of parents. But whether those reasons are decisive will be highly sensitive to
the particular circumstances the parents and child are in. As a result, it is far
harder to be confident that, in general, parents that have been keeping *the secret* should now disclose it. The details of their situation will really matter. But
even if some parents are right to continue keeping *the secret*, my argument
shows that it is still morally problematic both to have kept it in the first place
and to continue keeping it.

1. The standard arguments for disclosure

As I mentioned at the outset, the conclusion I'm arguing for is in line with
current recommendations that parents disclose to their children that they
are donor-conceived. But the argument I make for disclosure is novel. To see
why, let's briefly consider three standard arguments for disclosure.[7]

The first maintains that having genetic knowledge—which is to say, knowledge of who one's genetic progenitors are—is profoundly important for one's
sense of self.[8] According to this view, healthy identity formation depends on
knowing one's genetic origins. If that were true, then we would have a solid
rationale for disclosure for the simple reason that there's no plausible way for
a donor-conceived person to have genetic knowledge without knowing they
are donor-conceived. For reasons that will emerge in the coming chapters,
I am skeptical of claims about the profound importance of genetic knowledge for identity formation. So, I will not build a case for disclosure on it.

A second argument for disclosure points to the medical reasons for doing
so. If you do not even know that you are donor-conceived, then you will proceed through the world with a false picture of your family and medical history. You may think you are genetically prone to conditions that you are not,
in fact, genetically prone to. Conversely, you might be genetically prone to

---

[6] I say more about this prospect below (pp. 50–51).

[7] The three views I discuss are slight variants on the three De Melo-Martín discusses in Inmaculada De Melo-Martín, "The Ethics of Anonymous Gamete Donation: Is There a Right to Know One's Genetic Origins?," *Hastings Center Report* 44, no. 2 (2014): 28–35. She is interested in views that are meant to establish that people have a right to know who their genetic progenitors are. I'm interested in views that are meant to establish the more minimal claim that donor-conceived people have a right to know *that* they are donor-conceived.

[8] J. David Velleman, "The Gift of Life," *Philosophy & Public Affairs* 36, no. 3 (2008): 245–66; J. David Velleman, "Family History," *Philosophical Papers* 34, no. 3 (2005): 357–78.

conditions that you don't think you are genetically prone to. Whether or not there are strong medical reasons to know the *identity* of your donor, there are, according to this view, strong medical reasons to at least know *that* you are donor-conceived. I'll call this the Medical Disclosure argument.[9]

A third argument for disclosure points to the purported harm that keeping *the secret* can do to family members and overall family functioning.[10] I'll call this the Harmful Secrets argument. The most obvious concern on this front is that secrets are very hard to keep. The truth will often come out in less than ideal ways. For example, parents of donor-conceived children who do not intend to disclose to their child often tell other people, with the result that some donor-conceived people find out by accident from those other people.[11] Other times, *the secret* comes out after years and years of being kept, after years and years of child believing that their social parents are their genetic parents. Oftentimes in these cases, the child experiences considerable shock and dismay. Whatever bonds of trust existed between parents and child can be irrevocably severed. The children often feel betrayed.[12]

The difficulty of keeping *the secret* is increasingly acute in a world where information about one's genetic history is readily and cheaply available. As McGee, Brakman, and Gurmankin put it, secrecy "may well become a difficult struggle for an impossible result."[13] So parents who keep *the secret* should not be confident they can avoid the harmful effects of the truth coming out after many years.

But even when *the secret* never explicitly comes out, there is, according to the Harmful Secrets argument, potential for harm. The stress that comes with

---

[9] For an articulation of this view. see John B. Appleby, Lucy Blake, and Tabitha Freeman, "Is Disclosure in the Best Interests of Children Conceived by Donation?," *Reproductive donation.* (Cambridge: Cambridge University Press, 2012), 231–249.

[10] McGee, Brakman, and Gurmankin, "Gamete Donation and Anonymity" have an overview of the findings about the harm of keeping secrets in adoption. Paul and Berger find that there is an "inverse relationship between topic avoidance and family functioning." Marilyn S. Paul and Roni Berger, "Topic Avoidance and Family Functioning in Families Conceived with Donor Insemination," *Human Reproduction* 22, no. 9 (September 1, 2007): 2569, https://doi.org/10.1093/humrep/dem174. For a brief discussion of the "family therapy perspective" on keeping secrets see Golombok, *Modern Families,* 94–95.

[11] McGee et al. note, "In over half the studied cases where parents have reported their own choice not to tell the child of the use of donor gametes, other relatives or friends were told." McGee, Brakman, and Gurmankin, "Gamete Donation and Anonymity," 2033. In support of this contention they cite Susan C. Klock and Donald Maier, "Psychological Factors Related to Donor Insemination," *Fertility and Sterility* 56, no. 3 (September 1, 1991): 489–95. In the study of Swedish parents cited above, half of parents that had not told their child had told someone else: Lalos, Gottlieb, and Lalos, "Legislated Right for Donor-Insemination Children to Know Their Genetic Origin," 1759.

[12] Diane Ehrensaft, *Mommies, Daddies, Donors, Surrogates: Answering Tough Questions and Building Strong Families* (New York: Guilford Press, 2005), 156.

[13] McGee, Brakman, and Gurmankin, "Gamete Donation and Anonymity," 2033.

keeping the secret can be considerable. As one parent of adopted children put it to me, "You're constantly going to feel like you're lying. It's going to come up again and again," not just in conversations with the child, but with other people as well who make assumptions.[14] So keeping *the secret* is harmful to the parents who keep it, quite apart from whether it affects their child.

In all likelihood, however, it will affect the child and, more generally, overall family functioning. This is both because stress in parents is correlated with worse family functioning and also because the source of the stress plausibly effects, in ways subtle and not, how the parents interact with the child. Donor-conceived people who find our later in life report "knowing" or sensing that there was something amiss about their family situation, something that was left unsaid.[15] As Diane Ehrensaft puts it, "Children often sense secrets . . . and never feel fully accepted by the family if they suspect there is something about them nobody is talking about."[16] This sentiment is powerfully expressed by Shapiro, who writes, "All my life I had known there was a secret. What I hadn't known: the secret was me."[17]

Admittedly, we need to be careful with first-person accounts of "always knowing." It could be that people tell themselves "just so" stories about various normal and nearly universal childhood feelings and experiences in light of learning they are donor-conceived. Even so, we should be equally careful about giving no weight to these accounts. The view we are considering now—that even if *the secret* never explicitly comes out, it often does so implicitly—identifies a plausible mechanism by which a donor-conceived person comes to know, or suspect, that things are not quite as they seem when it comes to the nature of their family.

The Harmful Secrets argument posits a contingent, causal relationship between keeping *the secret* and the harms that can result. So it is not inevitable that keeping *the secret* will, as Ehrensaft puts it, engender "fissures and festering wounds."[18] In fact, talk of "fissures and festering wounds" outruns the available evidence on the harms of non-disclosure. Golombok claims that "the earlier children are told, the better the outcomes, and that discovering one's donor conception later in life may cause psychological harm." But, she says, "[i]t is important to emphasize . . . that the less positive findings for

---

[14] Personal correspondence. Used with permission.

[15] This is a theme throughout Dani Shapiro, *Inheritance: A Memoir of Genealogy, Paternity, and Love* (New York: Anchor, 2020).

[16] Ehrensaft, *Mommies, Daddies, Donors, Surrogates*, 156.

[17] Shapiro, *Inheritance*, 35.

[18] Ehrensaft, *Mommies, Daddies, Donors, Surrogates*, 155.

non-disclosing families did not represent clinical problems but fell within the range of normal."[19] Of course we don't know what will happen in these families if disclosure occurs. And there is no doubt that many donor-conceived people who only found out later in life that they are donor-conceived feel profoundly wronged by their social parents, as evidenced by the following reactions from two participants in a study on disclosure:[20]

I felt as if everybody had lied to me.
Shock, absolute disbelief, felt I'd been betrayed and lied to all my life.[21]

As the authors of this study note:

The respondents were frequently more concerned about prior parental deception than by their parents' use of donor conception. For some respondents this created relationship problems with their parents (especially mothers) and wider family, trust issues and deep feelings of anger and resentment.[22]

2. The Intimacy argument: an introduction

I believe that both the Medical Disclosure and Harmful Secrets arguments— each on its own, but certainly taken together—generally provide a decisive reason to disclose. I am on board, then, with the consensus view.[23] But I think

---

[19] Susan Golombok, "Disclosure and Donor-Conceived Children," *Human Reproduction* 32, no. 7 (2017): 1532.

[20] See Amanda J. Turner and Adrian Coyle, "What Does It Mean to Be a Donor Offspring? The Identity Experiences of Adults Conceived by Donor Insemination and the Implications for Counselling and Therapy," *Human Reproduction* 15, no. 9 (2000): 2041–51. For a strong first-person account of the feelings of betrayal that keeping the secret can engender, see Bill Cordray's contribution in Juliet Ruth Guichon, Ian Mitchell, and Michelle Giroux, eds., *The Right to Know One's Origins: Assisted Human Reproduction and the Best Interests of Children* (Brussels: ASP, 2012). Similar sentiments were also very clearly on display in the bulk of the crowd (many of whom were donor-conceived people who found out later in life) at the Ethics of Gamete Donation conference at NYU in May 2018.

[21] Lucy Frith et al., "Secrets and Disclosure in Donor Conception," *Sociology of Health & Illness* 40, no. 1 (2018): 7. The first quotation is from a conceived person who found out at 27. The second is from a donor-conceived person who found out at 38.

[22] Frith et al., "Secrets and Disclosure in Donor Conception," 7.

[23] Not everyone is. Inmaculada De Melo-Martín has argued that knowing one's family medical history is not as medically important as it is typically taken to be. However, she seems to admit that it is medically important to know *whether* one is donor-conceived: Melo-Martín, "The Ethics of Anonymous Gamete Donation," 32. For the contrary view, see Guido Pennings, "Disclosure of Donor Conception, Age of Disclosure and the Well-Being of Donor Offspring," *Human Reproduction* 32, no. 5 (May 1, 2017): 969–73. Pennings has argued that "there is little or no evidence one way

there is another kind of argument to be made for disclosure. The Medical Disclosure and Harmful Secrets arguments posit what we might call indirect harms of keeping *the secret*. In other words, they identify harms that are downstream from keeping *the secret*, harms that may (or may not) be realized. The argument I will make points to a different kind of harm that comes with keeping *the secret*.

To start, suppose that there were no negative medical consequences of disclosure. And suppose further that parents could keep *the secret* perfectly: not only would it never come out, but the child would never "sense" that there was something about her origins that she was not being told. Nor would anyone experience any of the subtler harms of keeping *the secret* (parental stress, family stress, *etc.*). The question we are left with is this: Would it then be acceptable for parents to keep *the secret*?

The answer, I will argue, is no (at least not normally). This is because keeping *the secret* directly harms the parent-child relationship. It damages the parent-child relationship insofar as it violates the norms of that relationship. Unlike the Harmful Secrets and Medical Disclosure arguments, my argument—which I call the Intimacy argument—doesn't depend on empirical claims about the contingent, downstream effects of keeping *the secret*. Rather, it argues from plausible assumptions about the nature of intimate relationships to the conclusion that keeping *the secret* constitutes a harm to the parent-child relationship. To borrow a metaphor from Shapiro, *the secret* corrodes the parent-child relationship all on its own, quite apart from whether it manifests in other ways.

or the other" about the negative consequences of non-disclosure. As a result, Pennings concludes that people should either avoid making a recommendation regarding disclosure or "state that all directions are equally good." He is aware, however, that there are other possible arguments for disclosure that are based, as he puts it, on "moral convictions" (972) or "implicit moral premises" (969) and not "science or evidence." I reject the implicit contrasts Pennings makes (between, for example, views based on evidence and moral convictions) and rather think all the views on offer are moral arguments for (or against) disclosure. But he is right that the Medical Disclosure and Harmful Secrets views depend on empirical claims about the downstream effects of non-disclosure, while other moral arguments—namely, those that appeal to "implicit moral premises"—do not. In the rest of this chapter, I make one of those arguments, although I try to leave none of the premises implicit. For responses to Pennings' critique of the Harmful Secrets view, see Marilyn Crawshaw et al., "Disclosure and Donor-Conceived Children," *Human Reproduction* 32, no. 7 (July 1, 2017): 1535–36. Golombok, "Disclosure and Donor-Conceived Children," 1532–36.

2.1. Is *the secret* really a secret? (Yes.)

Before turning to my argument, however, I want to defend my use of the term "the secret" to refer to parents not disclosing to their child that he is donor-conceived. Is non-disclosure the same as keeping a secret from the child? Not everyone thinks so. Iain Walker and Pia Broderick claim:

> Secrecy is a label borrowed from the area of family therapy and used by the mental health professionals involved in medically assisted reproduction. It is obviously an emotionally laden and strongly pejorative word. But what it refers to could equally well be described as maintaining privacy or confidentiality. [. . .] Using the label secrecy begs the question entirely: it assumes that which is to be demonstrated. The use of one label or another is a matter of fiat only; neither theory nor research can be used to justify either.[24]

Walker and Broderick are right about a number of things. Someone who is keeping a secret could aptly be described as maintaining privacy and confidentiality. Moreover, talk of keeping secrets in general, and certainly talk of keeping *the secret* as I've termed it, is emotionally laden. It suggests that there is something important behind the curtain.[25] In light of this, maybe we would do well to avoid "secret" talk *if* it really is just a matter of "fiat" which language we choose to describe non-disclosure, something that can be justified by "neither theory nor research."

But it is not just a matter of fiat which language we use here. There are good reasons for thinking of non-disclosure as keeping a secret. To get at them, consider Golombok's account of why parents choose not to disclose:

> When asked about their reasons for secrecy, parents of children born through egg, sperm or embryo donation have said they were worried their children would be upset, shocked and confused by the knowledge that they

---

[24] Iain Walker and Pia Broderick, "The Psychology of Assisted Reproduction—or Psychology Assisting Its Reproduction?," *Australian Psychologist* 34, no. 1 (1999): 31.

[25] I'm less convinced that it is a "strongly pejorative" word: it seems to me that friends, lovers, spouses, colleagues, government agencies, medical professionals keep secrets all the time and, rightly, no one bats an eye. But if marking something off as a "secret" does connote, at least sometimes, that it really *should* be disclosed (and again, a mark against this view is that information is classified as "secret" all the time where the suggestion is very much *not* that it should be disclosed), then we could put things in terms of keeping *confidences*. Everything I say about what I call *the secret* goes through if we call it *the confidence*.

were not genetically related to one parent (or both parents). The parents were also concerned about jeopardizing the positive relationship that existed between the non-genetic parent(s) and the child fearing that their child would no longer love the non-genetic parent(s) if they found out.[26]

These concerns are clearly on display in the following comments from parents of donor-conceived children:

"I wouldn't want her to feel that [father] wasn't her Dad."[27]

"I don't know how we're going to solve this problem [of not having disclosed] later . . . I'm afraid of losing my children, I'm not their father. I'm not the real one . . ."[28]

"X (the husband) doesn't want to . . . he's afraid the children will shun him, that something will be ruined as they have always believed something else . . ."[29]

"I'm old fashioned. We see it like this—what difference does it make? I can't see that it would make anything better. . . . [I]t could have the opposite effect . . . and I wouldn't be a dad anymore . . ."[30]

The takeaway here is that the central reason parents tend not to disclose is precisely that they worry the child will see the information as significant or important.[31] This feature of the situation makes non-disclosure different from many other facts about the child's conception that parents don't share. There are lots of things parents don't tell their children about the circumstances of their child's conception because the parents think they just aren't that important and so probably never even think about them. Or, if they do think about them, they don't see any reason why they should be shared. In these cases,

---

[26] Golombok, *Modern Families*, 99.

[27] Tabitha Freeman et al., "Disclosure of Sperm Donation: A Comparison between Solo Mother and Two-Parent Families with Identifiable Donors," *Reproductive Biomedicine Online* 33, no. 5 (2016): 597, square parentheses in the original.

[28] Lalos, Gottlieb, and Lalos, "Legislated Right for Donor-Insemination Children to Know Their Genetic Origin," 1763.

[29] Lalos, Gottlieb, and Lalos, "Legislated Right for Donor-Insemination Children to Know Their Genetic Origin," 1764.

[30] Lalos, Gottlieb, and Lalos, "Legislated Right for Donor-Insemination Children to Know Their Genetic Origin," 1764.

[31] Another common reason is that people worry that *other* people will see it as significant and in a way that will lead them to treat the child differently. I discuss this concern below (pp. 50–51).

non-disclosure—if we want to call it that—is not tantamount to keeping a secret precisely because there is no assumed significance to the information.

Not telling one's child she is donor-conceived is different. Even if the fact that the child is donor-conceived is truly a matter of indifference to the parents, which it probably isn't, the parents think that *the child* will see it as significant *and this is precisely why they do not disclose.*[32] And if anything counts as keeping a secret from another person, it is withholding information from them precisely because you think they will see the information as significant. For the most part, then, parents of donor-conceived children who do not disclose are keeping a secret from their child. Using the term is neither unjustified nor a matter of fiat.

2.2. Is keeping the secret deceptive? (Almost always yes.)

So not telling one's child that they are donor-conceived is keeping a secret from them. But is it deceptive? Clearly it is, if it involves baldly lying to the child about their genetic origins. But not all secret keeping, either in general or in the case of keeping *the secret*, involves lying. The situation might never arise where the parents of a donor-conceived person need to guard *the secret* with a lie. As a result, if keeping *the secret* is deceptive, it is not because it necessarily involves lying.

There is also no necessary connection between keeping a secret from someone and deceiving that person. I keep details of my financial situation secret from most people, but I do not thereby deceive my friends about my finances. But suppose—without ever explicitly lying—I present myself as relatively poor when, in fact, I am extremely well-off: I buy only second-hand clothes, note the rising cost of basic goods, worry about the state of the economy, *etc.* And suppose I do all this knowing that this will lead my friends to believe I am less well-off than I am. Indeed, suppose this is *why* I do it. My friends are not particularly well-off and I'm worried about how they'll treat me if they realize I have a lot of money. Although I never lie to them, I present

---

[32] This is not to say that parents would disclose if they really believed that the information would be seen as irrelevant by the child, as neither interesting nor important. But now the reason for non-disclosure would be totally different, so much so that it's not clear that we should even call it "non-disclosure". There would, in a sense, be nothing to disclose, in much the same way that parents not telling their child who was on the cover of *TV Guide* the week they were conceived isn't a case of *non-disclosure*. It's just not something anyone cares about.

myself in a way that foreseeably leads them to false beliefs. In doing so, I deceive my friends.

Keeping *the secret* is akin to deceiving my friends about my financial security. If parents keep *the secret*, then the child will foreseeably be very likely to believe that both of his parents are his genetic parents. Why? Because they will have been given no indication that how they came to be departs from what we might call the "default story" of how families are formed. We all know the default story: babies are conceived when a man and a woman who love each other have sex for the purpose of creating a baby. Families—where children are the genetic offspring of the people that raise them—are the result of this process. But we also all know this is very often *not* how families are made. And no doubt many people make clear to their children that the default story doesn't apply to all families. But usually such clarity comes in the form of pointing to *exceptions* to the default story, a move that has the effect of foregrounding the default story as the *default*.[33]

Now many children will never subscribe to the default story of how they (and their family) came to be because their family form won't allow for it. Children of single parents or lesbian or gay parents will realize as they grow up that the default is not—could not be—their family's story. But for that very reason, keeping *the secret* is not a live option in these families.[34] It is only an option in those families that—by all appearances—could have been formed according to the default story. And parents that keep *the secret* are taking advantage of exactly that feature of their family form. They are, in effect, passing as a family made according to the default story. And that will foreseeably lead the child to believe her parents are her genetic parents *precisely because that is the default story*. There is a self-reinforcing dynamic at play. Keeping *the secret* allows the default story to take hold in the child's mind in the first place. This, in turn, makes it easier to keep *the secret* since the default story effectively prevents the question of one's genetic origins from arising in the first place.

But is keeping *the secret* deceptive? Certainly it is if parents *intend* to use the availability of the default story to induce their child to believe that both her parents are her genetic progenitors. And the quotations we saw earlier from parents who have not disclosed strongly suggest that this is often the

---

[33] An exception to this is Cory Silverberg, *What Makes a Baby* (New York: Seven Stories Press, 2013).

[34] Well, it is more viable in the case of a single parent who needn't disclose that the child was donor-conceived.

intention. There is palpable anxiety that the child's attachment to the non-genetic parent will disappear if the child finds out she is donor-conceived.[35] And so the goal is to ensure that the child never comes to realize that one, or both, parents are not her genetic progenitors. The goal is to pass as a "normal" family, one that was formed according to the default story.

One might argue that even here the parents are not deceiving the child because they are merely(!) *allowing* their child to be deceived by circumstances. But this is implausible. The parents are not bystanders to the default story taking hold, but active and knowing participants. They have their role to play, namely as parents that fit into the default story. In other words, they are part of the story. And they know it. They are involved in the deception and not just allowing it to happen.

The same is true of parents who initially intended to disclose, but then don't. So long as they do not disclose they knowingly, even if in some sense unwillingly, play the role assigned them by the default story (i.e. that of parent as genetic progenitor). They may not have intended to deceive, but they are now playing a part in the ongoing deception of their child. They may still intend to disclose, but to the extent they fail to do so, they are buying time by partaking in the deception.

Is there a way to keep *the secret* without deception? Maybe. Suppose a set of parents were extremely clear from the start that there is no one way to make a family. Rather than using a story that foregrounds the default story, they might use a story that goes out of its way to emphasize the different ways families come to be. We can imagine further that the parents themselves make a point of noting that one should never make assumptions about how a family came to be. Nonetheless, they never disclose to their child that she is donor-conceived.

Now it will be very hard to keep *the secret* in these circumstances. The parents' approach is sure to invite queries from the child about how *she* specifically came to be. But let's imagine the child is especially incurious and so never asks about how she specifically came to be. In this implausible case, the parents might non-deceptively keep *the secret*. But the implausibility of the example is its point. Real-world examples of keeping *the secret* just don't (and won't) work like this. In the real world, keeping *the secret* is deceptive.

---

[35] One thing that is striking about the quotations is the extent to which the parents—especially the fathers—buy into a biogenetic conception of parenthood. They worry that the child will *discover* that one parent is not the "real" parent, as though genetic relatedness provides the grounds of normative parenthood.

3. The Intimacy argument explained

Keeping *the secret* is more or less always deceptive. I assume most people will think that counts as a mark against it. But maybe it's not a serious mark. After all, parents deceive their kids all the time in ways that most people think are acceptable. Santa Claus, the Easter Bunny, and the Tooth Fairy are obvious examples. But there are also all kinds of everyday deceptions parents engage in: telling a younger sibling that his older sister is also going to bed now even though she will actually be staying up longer; or telling a child "maybe" when you know full well the answer is "never";[36] or telling a child that their artwork is "really good" when it's actually garbage (and destined for the garbage).[37]

Some may think that these deceptions are unjustified, that it is almost always wrong to deceive one's child. If that's you, then the lesson is not that the deception of keeping *the secret* is justified, but rather that all the other ways in which parents deceive their children are unjustified. But perhaps instead the examples of common forms of parental deception strike you as morally mundane. And perhaps you're not sure just how problematic the deception of keeping *the secret* is. Maybe you're thinking it really isn't so different from morally mundane deceptions.

It is. Recall that what is being kept secret has assumed significance: parents assume their child will think the fact that they are donor-conceived will matter to them profoundly. Right away, this separates the deception of non-disclosure from more mundane deceptions. The latter are usually geared to smoothing over, or moving past, a potentially fraught moment (e.g. bedtime). There is no assumption that the information that is withheld will have lifelong significance. So, on the face of it, the deception of keeping *the secret* is not of a piece with mundane parental deception.

---

[36] Mind you, this move has a short shelf life.
[37] A special thanks to Kaethe Schwehn for a litany of personal examples:

"You can be whatever you want to be when you grow up."
"Being good at math is just about working hard."
"We don't care what grades/test scores you get, as long as you're doing the best you can."
"Mommy isn't using a plastic kiddie cup to bring home the remainder of her martini from the restaurant. Stop imagining things."
"I'd love to know more about the parts of the violin. Please tell me!"
"You will be stronger/faster/smarter/have bigger boobs if you eat the goddamn butternut squash soup."
"All families have strict rules about something, it's just not always the same thing."
"We will come up to bed in 20 minutes."
"Mommy is too tired to play UNO."
"I really have to send this e-mail right now and thus cannot do X or Y or Z."

But it still might not be obvious why we should care about this deception if we take seriously the stipulation I made earlier, namely that the secret can be perfectly kept and has no medical implications. If there are no negative psychological or medical repercussions of keeping *the secret*, then what's the problem?

A full answer to that question would require a deep dive into the nature of harm and wrongs. But let's stay out of those waters. Instead, I will argue that keeping the secret violates norms of intimacy by creating *distance* between parents and children that is at odds with the demands of intimacy in the parent-child relationship. It prevents a degree of closeness that ought to be present in the parent-child relationship. Before explaining why that is, we need to be clear about just what my claim is. My claim is not that keeping *the secret* creates *felt* distance in the parent-child relationship. That would amount to a restatement of the Harmful Secrets view. My claim, rather, is that keeping *the secret* directly introduces a kind of distance into the relationship that should not be there, whether it is "felt" by any of the parties or not.

But then what does talk of "distance" and "closeness" mean in this context if they are not to be explained in terms of the knock-on experienced effects of keeping *the secret*? To answer that question, consider some near-platitudes about what it means to be close to someone. To be close to someone is to know her well, to know what matters to her and why (at least to some extent); it is to care about what she cares about, partly *because* she cares about it; it is to knowingly share, at least to some extent, concerns or cares, i.e. for the other person's cares to be one's own and vice versa; it is to care about how the person's life goes for their own sake; and, most important for our purposes, it is to trust that person both as a giver and a receiver of personally important information.[38]

Relationships can be close in some ways, but not others. I might know a lot about what matters to you, but not share some of your deepest concerns or cares; or I might care a tremendous amount about what happens to you, but not know very much about what matters to you and why; I might share a lot of your concerns and cares, but not trust you much at all with my personally important information. In all these cases, we are not as close as we might be.

---

[38] Kyla Ebels-Duggan, "Against Beneficence: A Normative Account of Love," *Ethics* 119, no. 1 (2008): 142–70. Ebels-Duggan doesn't put things in exactly these terms, preferring the Kantian notions of "sharing ends" and granting one's beloved certain kinds of authority ("selection authority" and "authority in judgment"). The last item on my list of the marks of a loving relationship, namely to trust the other person both as a giver and receiver of personally important information, could, I think, figure into an expanded account of the kind of authority lovers ought to grant each other,

Naturally, not all relationships should be close—distance is perfectly appropriate between colleagues, for example. But some relationships should be close because their value inheres, at least in part, in the fact that they are intimate (consider, for example, your dearest friendships). The parent-child relationship—especially before the child reaches full maturity and relative independence—is one such relationship. This means that parents should be wary of doing things that compromise the intimacy of the relationship.[39] And keeping *the secret*, I claim, is precisely one of those things that compromises the intimacy of the relationship.

The last feature of intimacy I noted above—trusting the other person to give and receive personally important information—is at odds with keeping *the secret*. The trust at issue here is not just about confidentiality, i.e. about whether the information will be shared more widely. It is, more fundamentally, about whether the information can be handled. I've put the point in the passive voice on purpose. Sometimes, the worry might be that the other person cannot handle the information. The worry is that the information will cause real harm—psychological or otherwise—to the other person and that is why you keep it a secret.[40] But other times, the worry is less about the harm it might cause the other person and more about the harm it might cause to your *relationship* with the person. The relationship, and not (just) the other person, cannot handle the information being disclosed and that is why you keep a secret.

When it comes to *the secret*, both worries about "handling" the information are in play. Parents worry about whether the news will cause distress for their child. But they also worry about what disclosure will do to their relationship with their child, all the more so if they have been keeping *the secret* for some time. Crucially, the issue here is not whether parents are justified in having these worries. The point is that their concern—justified or not—is,

---

although perhaps the kind of trust I mention here is implied by the kinds of authority Ebels-Duggan discusses. Crucially, Ebels-Duggan's account is about love between adults, not children and parents. As she rightly notes, the parent-child relationship permits a high degree of paternalism that would be thoroughly insulting in a relationship between adult lovers.

[39] For a discussion of the nature and value of intimacy between parents and children, see Harry Brighouse and Adam Swift, *Family Values: The Ethics of Parent-Child Relationships* (Princeton, NJ: Princeton University Press, 2014), chapter 4. Brighouse and Swift draw their inspiration from Ferdinand Schoeman, "Rights of Children, Rights of Parents, and the Moral Basis of the Family," *Ethics* 91, no. 1 (October 1, 1980): 6–19, https://doi.org/10.1086/292199.

[40] For a powerful account of this kind of calculation, see *This American Life*, "585: In Defense of Ignorance," December 14, 2017, https://www.thisamericanlife.org/585/transcript.

by itself, at odds with the kind of intimacy that should be present in the relationship. It evinces a lack of trust (justified or not) in both their child and their relationship with the child about whether either can bear the (assumed) weight of disclosure.

These concerns are amplified by the nature of *the secret*. To see why, consider another secret that someone in an intimate relationship might keep: suppose Amelia has a serious gambling problem and hasn't told her partner, Sharon, about it. One of Amelia's main worries about disclosing this secret is that it will damage her relationship with Sharon. To that extent, Amelia's worries about telling Sharon about her gambling problem is the same as the parents' worries about disclosing to their child that they are donor-conceived.

But notice this difference: Amelia's secret is not about her relationship with Sharon. It's about her gambling. *The secret*, on the other hand, is precisely about the very relationship that parents worry is threatened by disclosure. More than that, it is about the *grounds* of the relationship between the parents and their child. To see what I mean by that, imagine Amelia is keeping another secret from Sharon. Sharon believes that her meeting Amelia was entirely serendipitous: they happened to sit next to each other in class one day back in college and, *voilà*, a great love was born. What Sharon doesn't know is that Amelia noticed Sharon well before Sharon noticed her. Amelia asked Melvin, the person who normally sat next to Sharon in class, to not occupy his usual seat the day Amelia and Sharon met precisely so Amelia could "just happen" to sit next to Amelia. Amelia has a secret about the cause of her relationship with Sharon. But Amelia and Sharon's differing beliefs about how they met—whether it was serendipity or romantic cunning—plays no role in their understanding of what currently grounds their relationship. If we were to ask each of them, "What makes Amelia/Sharon your life partner?" they would both say something like "Because we love each other and are committed to each other." How they met is part of the causal story of why they are partners. But the basis, or grounds, of their relationship—the thing that makes them partners in an ongoing way—is something else altogether: it is their continuing concern and care for each other. To put it differently, how they met was the occasion for their partnership, but it plays no role in their understanding of what currently sustains it.

The secret is not like this. A child who does not know he was donor-conceived not only has a different conception of what caused these people—whoever they are—to be his parents, but also (in all likelihood) a different understanding of what *now* binds them together as parents and child. In other words, the relationship proceeds under false pretenses about the nature of the ongoing relationship itself. Now, it does not proceed under entirely false pretenses. The parents might say, "Our loving commitment to raising this child is what matters. That, and not genetic relatedness, is what binds us together as parents and child." That is surely true and, in my view, it is the most important part of the story of what binds people together as parents and children. But it is also true that when parents keep *the secret*, the child comes to think that at least *part* of the basis for why these people are her parents—why they, and not others, are the ones who are lovingly raising her—is that she is their genetic offspring. Why? Because of the default story, which functions to explain why these particular people are her parents. Keeping *the secret*, then, ensures a mismatch between the parents and child about the very basis of their intimate relationship. *The secret* builds into the very structure of the relationship.

Why think that this distance is a threat to the intimacy of the relationship? One possible answer is that *any* distance in a relationship is at odds with intimacy. Maybe that's true. But as I already noted above, a lack of intimacy is hardly a failing when it comes to many kinds of relationships. It would be strange and inappropriate if my relationship with a colleague, considered simply as a colleague, were as intimate as a relationship can be! The colleague relationship *should* have all kinds of distance built into it. So merely noting that something compromises the intimacy of a relationship does not show that there's anything wrong with it.

I've already noted that the parent-child relationship is one that should be highly intimate, that the value of the relationship inheres in large part from the intimacy it embodies (when it is going well). But even those relationships that we typically think of as intimate should have some distance. And this is certainly true of the parent-child relationship. A parent who shares *everything* with their child—all their anxieties, hardships, hopes, and passions—oversteps. They burden their child. Likewise, children—particularly adult children, but also to some extent young children—should have interests, hopes, anxieties, and passions that they don't share with their parents. In other words, the parent-child relationship should be not maximally intimate. Some amount of distance is proper to the relationship.

The question, then, is this: Is the distance introduced by *the secret* at odds with the intimacy that is proper to the parent-child relationship? I think it is. Rather than attempt to give a general account of what degree of intimacy is proper to the parent-child relationship, let me offer two considerations in support of my claim.

First, recall a point I made above: *the secret* is not just about the cause of the parent-child relationship, but also its ground. It effectively ensures—and indeed often aims for the result—that the child misunderstands the basis of the ongoing parent-child relationship. Perhaps it is proper to *every* kind of relationship that the parties in it are not substantially misaligned in their understanding of the grounds of the relationship. But I don't need to invoke such a strong principle for my purposes. For surely it is proper to *intimate* relationships. In other words, intimate relationships are compromised to the extent that the people in the relationship have substantially different understandings of the grounds of the relationship and all the more so if one party in the relationship is intentionally inculcating the misunderstanding in another.

The second reason[41] that keeping *the secret* is at odds with the intimacy proper to the parent-child relationship appeals to a plausible corollary of the near-platitudes about closeness I mentioned earlier: being close to another person involves sharing information about the other person that you have reason to believe will be meaningful to them. This is part of being close to another person, since it involves both taking seriously the other person's view of what is (likely to be) meaningful to them *and* trusting their ability to handle it. There is probably no general answer as to how and when one should share such information. And even if we focus on the specific information we are interested in here—namely that one's child is donor-conceived—just how and when one should share the information is none too clear. Clearly, it would be foolish to think that a young child could understand, let alone handle, full-blown information about the fact that they are donor-conceived.[42] But even if getting the precise timing and telling right is difficult, the point is that *never* telling is at odds with the demands of parent-child intimacy.

---

[41] For which I am indebted to Andrée-Anne Cormier.

[42] As Hertz and Nelson put it, "For very young children, the 'donor' is a hollow concept" and donor conception needs to be explained again and again in age-appropriate terms. One point that emerges from their discussion is that disclosure needs to happen again and again as children get older and are able to better understand what donor conception is:

> Parents frequently told us that they had talked about the donor from the moment a child was born; many told us they had read from the available children's books about donor conception. They thought their children fully understood what they needed to know. But even clever young children like Haley and Olivia [two of the participants in the authors' fieldwork] confessed that it was a long time before they fully understood what a donor was and how donor conception came about.

Rosanna Hertz and Margaret K. Nelson, *Random Families: Genetic Strangers, Sperm Donor Siblings, and the Creation of New Kin* (New York: Oxford University Press, 2018), 33–35.

Both of these reasons generate a strong presumption against keeping *the secret*. But it is only a presumption. Every intimate relationship contains secrets. And some intimate relationships are not only built, but depend for their continued existence, on secrets. Secrets in intimate relationships— including *the secret*—might be highly instrumentally valuable, so much so that it would be a mistake to reveal them. But the presumption is that such secrets should not be kept. Moreover, even when the totality of considerations suggests that they should, the presence of such secrets counts against the quality of the relationship if keeping them is at odds with the intimacy proper to the relationship. This is especially true when the secrets are about the grounds of the relationship itself. And that is precisely the case with *the secret*.

4. Tying it all together

I have argued that keeping *the secret* is problematic because it directly harms the parent-child relationship by compromising the intimacy that is proper to the relationship. But what is the weight of this view when thinking about whether parents should disclose? I think it is quite weighty inasmuch as it cuts to the heart of what makes for a good parent-child relationship. Parents who keep *the secret* are doing something substantially wrong.

But whether keeping *the secret* is usually wrong all things considered will depend on what else is at stake. There would be strong reason to keep *the secret* if we had good reason to think that whatever harm to intimacy comes with keeping it is less than the harm to the child-parent relationship that results from disclosing.

At this point, it is crucial to bear in mind the distinction we made at the start of the chapter between parents who wonder about whether to keep *the secret* in the first place versus those who are wondering about whether to continue keeping it. Finding out—particularly later in life—that one is donor-conceived can cause a serious rupture between child and parents if the latter have been keeping *the secret*. But that's not the kind of case we should focus on. Instead, the question is whether there are significant downsides to a donor-conceived person having always known they are donor-conceived.

The available evidence suggests that the answer is "no." The evidence from adoption is quite clear, both with respect to the harms of late disclosure and the benefits of early disclosure. So-called Late Discovery Adoptees are more likely to experience "feelings of betrayal, loss of trust, and difficulty forgiving."[43] They also report "more distress and lower life satisfaction."[44] On the other side, adoptees who were told when they were very young

[a]ppreciated the fact that their adoptive parents had told them about the adoption when they were quite young, and this often helped the adoptee's sense of identity and belonging. For example, some adoptees indicated that being told early in life meant that adoption was not an issue, they always felt that they belonged, and that there was no sense of confusion later.[45]

There is less evidence when it comes to effects of early disclosure in families with donor-conceived children. However, Golombok reports:

In a study of the thoughts and feelings of adolescents who had grown up with the knowledge that they were donor-conceived, the majority reported feeling comfortable about their donor conception and felt that learning about their donor conception had not had a negative impact on their relationship with their parents.[46]

Moreover, more than one study shows that parents "do not appear to regret telling their children they were donor-conceived."[47] But what is generally true is not universally true. Particular intended parents might have good reason to think that *their* parent-child relationship will suffer if they disclose. But in general, those kinds of worries don't justify keeping *the secret*.

While concerns about the parent-child relationship might be the main reason people tend to not disclose, it is not the only one. Another common reason is that parents are concerned about how other people—including

[43] Amanda L. Baden et al., "Delaying Adoption Disclosure: A Survey of Late Discovery Adoptees," *Journal of Family Issues*, May 14, 2019, 1159.

[44] Baden et al., "Delaying Adoption Disclosure," 1154.

[45] N. L. Passmore, A. R. Foulstone, and J.A. Feeney, "Openness and Secrecy in Adoptive Families and Possible Effects on the Interpersonal Relationships of Adult Adoptees.," in *Relationships—Near and Far: Proceedings of the APS Psychology of Relationships Interest Group 6th Annual Conference*, ed. Barry J. Fallon (Melbourne: Australian Psychological Society, n.d.), 5.

[46] Golombok, *Modern Families*, 105.

[47] Golombok, *Modern Families*, 105. She appeals to the following studies: F. Lindblad, C. Gottlieb, and O. Lalos, "To Tell or Not to Tell: What Parents Think about Telling Their Children That They Were Born Following Donor Insemination," *Journal of Psychosomatic Obstetrics & Gynecology* 21, no. 4 (2000): 193–203; Kirstin MacDougall et al., "Strategies for Disclosure: How Parents Approach Telling Their Children That They Were Conceived with Donor Gametes," *Fertility and Sterility* 87, no. 3 (2007): 524–33; Joanna E. Scheib, Maura Riordan, and Susan Rubin, "Choosing Identity-Release

extended family—will treat their child.[48] It is very hard to say whether such concerns are well founded. While some people's concerns might be over-blown, others' surely are not. For the latter group, whatever intrinsic loss of intimacy comes with keeping *the secret* might be worth the gain in commu-nity or (extended) family cohesiveness.

At this point, I want to emphasize two points that might have fallen out of view. The first has to do with why we're even considering the Intimacy ar-gument. It is not meant to justify disclosure on its own, but rather to sit on the scale alongside the Medical Disclosure and Harmful Secrets arguments, which (particularly taken together) make a strong case for disclosure. The point of giving the Intimacy argument was to get at another weighty reason for disclosure that is easy to overlook precisely because of the force of the two standard arguments.[49] But in thinking about whether, overall, people should disclose, we need to consider not only the loss of intimacy but also the potential downstream harms that come with non-disclosure. When we do that, it is safe to conclude that there is a very strong presumption in favor of disclosing.

It is still just a presumption, though. And that is the second point to keep in mind. The conclusion that parents should disclose is general, not uni-versal. Particular parents might find themselves in situations where there is overwhelmingly good reason to keep *the secret*. Maybe disclosure will tear their family asunder. Maybe the child was conceived in circumstances where disclosure will lead to ostracization of the child or family. In cases like these, the balance of considerations might tip toward keeping *the secret* (although even here, parents need to consider the very real possibility that it will come out eventually).

Sperm Donors: The Parents' Perspective 13–18 Years Later," *Human Reproduction* 18, no. 5 (2003): 1115–27.

[48] Petra Nordqvist and Carol Smart, *Relative Strangers: Family Life, Genes and Donor Conception* (New York: Springer, 2014), 72–76; Lalos, Gottlieb, and Lalos, "Legislated Right for Donor-Insemination Children to Know Their Genetic Origin."

[49] Having said that, if someone thinks the reason I've identified is trifling, then there won't have been much point in bringing it into view. Compare: "Focusing on the need of the child drowning in the shallow pond when discussing why one is required to jump in to save him threatens to cover over *other* reasons why one should jump in. For example: getting your heart rate up is good for you and jumping into the pond will get your heart rate up! So that's a reason to jump in!" True enough. But this trifling reason is not worth discussing.

5. One more consideration: avoiding the "inevitable question"

By way of concluding, let's consider one more reason parents might want to keep *the secret*. Golombok reports that some parents who have not (yet) disclosed do not "know how to tell their children and, *as the donors were anonymous*, they were concerned about not being able to answer their child's inevitable question: 'If you are not my biological parent, then who is?' "[50]

The parents Golombok is talking about are already keeping *the secret*. For all the reasons we've covered, whether they should disclose if they cannot answer the inevitable question is (once again) hardly obvious. But we might ask whether the *prospect* of being unable to answer the inevitable question gives intended parents a weighty reason to keep *the secret* in the first place. Some intended parents—like those in France—face the prospect of not being able to answer the inevitable question whether they want to or not because they have no choice but to use anonymously donated gametes. But we are wondering about intended parents who do have a choice to use a non-anonymous donor. So our question is this: Does planning to use an anonymous donor give intended parents a weighty reason to keep *the secret* (given that they won't be able to answer the inevitable question)?

The answer depends in part on whether it is permissible to use an anonymous donor in the first place. If it's not, then *even if* using an anonymous donor gave parents a weighty reason to keep *the secret* in the first place, they effectively buy that reason by doing something wrong. So, keeping *the secret* would, once again, be morally fraught.

Whether it is permissible to use an anonymous donor is the topic of the next few chapters. But note: the proposal that it might be okay to keep *the secret* because you cannot answer the inevitable question presupposes that you have put your child in a bad spot. You have brought the pressing question "If you're not my biological parent, then who is?" to the fore without being able

---

[50] Golombok, *Modern Families*, 100, emphasis added. Worries about being able to answer the inevitable question naturally raise the question of whether intended parents should choose a *known* donor since using an open donor also means that parents will not be able to answer the inevitable question, at least for a while (assuming they told their child when the child was young). As Hertz and Nelson note, for children conceived with anonymous and open donors, "the donor remain[s] a mystery to be solved." Hertz and Nelson, *Random Families*, 35. I consider this line of thought in chapter 8.

to answer it. To claim that it is better to keep *the secret* in these circumstances is to acknowledge that there is something wrong with simultaneously *piquing* your child's interest in having an answer to the question and choosing, in advance, to not be able to answer it.

What this line of reasoning suggests is that disclosing to a child that they are donor-conceived probably does not *generate* an interest in knowing who one's genetic progenitor is but rather reveals to the child that *an interest they have always had but took to be fulfilled* has not, in fact, been fulfilled. Indeed, as we saw above one of the purposes of keeping *the secret* is to make the child believe their family is "normal," to lead them to think, "These are my parents *in the typical sense of the term.*" The purpose, in other words, is to make them think there is no open question.

It is possible that when someone learns she is donor-conceived it *generates* an interest in genetic knowledge that was not present before. But that seems a stretch. As we will see in the next chapter, the majority of donor-conceived people (who know they are donor-conceived) are interested in obtaining genetic knowledge. Suppose we pointed out to these people that prior to learning they were donor-conceived they expended no real energy in thinking about—let alone seeking out—who their genetic progenitors are. It seems unlikely they would say, "Yes, that's because I didn't care" rather than "Yes, that's because I didn't know I am donor-conceived." If that's right, then choosing to keep *the secret* because one plans to use an anonymous donor is not a way of avoiding frustrating the child's likely interest in having genetic knowledge. It is, rather, a way of hiding from the child that their interest is already being frustrated.

Is there something wrong with that, i.e. with frustrating an interest that the child is likely to have? And if so, is it *so* wrong that (normally) parents shouldn't use an anonymous donor in the first place? The answer to both questions, I will argue, is "yes." The point for now is that whether keeping *the secret* is justified because you plan to use an anonymous donor (and so won't be able to answer the inevitable question) depends on whether the prior decision to use an anonymous donor is justified. Worries about not being able to answer the inevitable question because you plan to use an anonymous donor do not generate a reason, let alone a decisive one, to keep *the secret*, unless there is some independent decisive reason to put yourself in the position where you cannot answer the inevitable question. If there is not—if, that is, intended parents should use open donors—then the worry about not being able to answer the inevitable question will not arise at all.[51] To the extent that it does, it is because the parents have already gone wrong (by using an anonymous donor). The work of the next three chapters is to show that, normally, they have.

---

[51] This is too strong. If parents use an open donor, they won't be able to answer the question right away. But they will be able to answer it eventually. This is the kind of point that might push some to wonder whether parents ought to use a known donor. See chapter 1 for my thoughts on this, as well as chapter 8.

3

The Significant Interest View

When I found out, I was not heartbroken or devastated (unlike
the popular belief), but I was more curious than anything else. 10
minutes after I found out, a dozen questions flowed out of my mouth
in less than a minute.

—A 13-year-old on his experience of learning he was
donor-conceived. From Vasanti Jadva et al., "The Experiences of
Adolescents and Adults Conceived by Sperm Donation," 2009

I think when people say "everyone" loves something, they're being
a little loose with the word "everyone." Everyone loves food and air.
And Matt Damon. But that's about it, probably. It's not a good feeling
when someone says "everyone," but they don't mean you. I guess
that's all I wanted to say.

—Gene, *Bob's Burgers,* season 8, episode 9, 2018

This chapter starts to answer the central question: Should intended parents
who plan to conceive with donated gametes use an open donor? As we saw
in chapter 1, the simplest reason to think the answer is "yes" is that having
genetic knowledge can be critically important for medical reasons. However,
stopping with the Medical Reasons view prevents us from considering the
deeper issues with donor conception that interest us. So a reformulated version of the central question is this: If there were *no* medical reasons to access
genetic knowledge, would there be reason(s) for intended parents to use an
open donor? The answer, I shall argue, is "yes."[1]

You might think answering "yes" depends on the idea that genetic
knowledge is profoundly important for people, that a life that lacks it is
impoverished. I'll say more about what this view amounts to below and then

---

[1] In chapter 6 I consider whether, in light of competing considerations, that reason is decisive.

Conceiving People. Daniel Groll, Oxford University Press. © Oxford University Press 2021.
DOI: 10.1093/oso/9780190063054.003.0003

a lot more in the next chapter. But the basic idea is that determining one's identity is fantastically hard to do without genetic knowledge. According to this view, genetic knowledge is a *profound prudential good* and people who lack it will have tremendous trouble figuring out who they are. I call this the Profound Prudential Good view.

Another way to make the case that intended parents should use an open donor appeals to the idea that people have a right to genetic knowledge.[2] There are two versions of this view.[3] The first is that people have a basic right to genetic knowledge. The second claims that people have a right to genetic knowledge because of a more general autonomy right to shape their identities as they see fit.

My argument depends neither on the claim that genetic knowledge is profoundly prudentially important nor on the claim that donor-conceived people have a right to genetic knowledge. Rather, it turns on general claims about (1) parents' obligations to help promote their children's well-being and (2) the connection between a person's well-being and the satisfaction of what I will call their "worthwhile significant subjective interests." To put my view (too) simply: the fact that a donor-conceived person is quite likely to be very interested in having genetic knowledge gives intended parents a weighty reason to use an open donor. This is because parents should promote their children's well-being *through* the satisfaction of their child's worthwhile significant subjective interests. I call this the Significant Interest view.

Though it will become clear as we proceed, I want to highlight a central feature of the Significant Interest view: it does not *directly* depend on claims about the value of genetic knowledge. Instead, most of the normative work in the argument depends on the premise that it matters that many donor-conceived people are subjectively interested in having genetic knowledge. In other words, the Significant Interest view turns on a claim about the need to take seriously the psychology of many donor-conceived people.

Admittedly, it does not turn only on that claim. I am committed to the idea that we should (normally) see a donor-conceived person's subjective interest in genetic knowledge as *worthwhile*. And this might lead to two closely related questions in the reader's mind. First, in admitting that a subjective interest in genetic knowledge is worthwhile, isn't the Significant Interest view

---

[2] The rights-based account is not at odds with the first approach. Indeed, one might use claims about the profound prudential importance of genetic knowledge to ground claims about a right to genetic knowledge.

[3] I said more about both in chapter 1.

a mere sideshow? In other words, if the Significant Interest view concedes that an interest in genetic knowledge is worthwhile, why not base the argument for using an open donor on *what makes the interest worthwhile,* and not the (supposedly) derivative fact that donor-conceived people tend to have a subjective interest in having genetic knowledge? I'll call this the Sideshow objection.

The second question is this: If the Significant Interest view concedes that the interest in genetic knowledge is worthwhile *and* claims that intended parents contribute to their child's well-being by giving them access to genetic knowledge, how is the Significant Interest view different from the Profound Prudential Good view?

I answer the second question in this chapter. Answering the first—and so the Sideshow objection—requires an account of why an interest in genetic knowledge is worthwhile. The full answer only comes in chapters 4 and 5, but I can give part of the response now. When I claim that a person's interest in genetic knowledge is (normally) worthwhile, I mean something very minimal: the interest is neither trivial (it not like an interest in counting blades of grass) nor morally problematic (it's not like an interest in torturing animals, say). This minimal sense in which the interest is worthwhile is all I need to get the Significant Interest view off the ground.[4] This gives me two responses to the Sideshow objection.

First, even if a direct positive account of the value of genetic knowledge *could* ground an argument for the conclusion that intended parents should use an open donor, there is still good reason for offering the Significant Interest view. Claims about the value of genetic knowledge are controversial. So too is the claim that intended parents should conceive with an open donor. If we can establish that conclusion by way of relatively uncontroversial premises—particularly without taking a stand on the value of genetic knowledge beyond claiming that an interest in it is worthwhile in my minimal sense—then that would be something! People might disagree about the nature and extent of genetic knowledge's value. But so long as people agree that people's interest in it clears a relatively low bar—it is neither trivial nor morally problematic—then the Significant Interest view succeeds.

The second response to the Sideshow objection is more direct. The Significant Interest view is not a sideshow to a more direct argument based

---

[4] Some might think the interest *is* morally problematic, while admitting it is not like an interest in watching dog fighting. I consider, and respond to, this objection in chapter 5.

on the value of genetic knowledge because there is no such plausible argument. The proper account of the value of genetic knowledge cannot, in my view, plausibly be deployed to show that intended parents should use an open donor. I argue for this claim in chapter 4, where I *do* offer a positive account of the value of genetic knowledge. The point here is just that the Significant Interest view is, as far as I'm concerned, the real deal: it provides the actual rationale for thinking that intended parents have a weighty reason to use an open donor.[5]

1. The Profound Prudential Good view

The Significant Interest view claims there is a connection between having genetic knowledge and well-being. The Profound Prudential Good view also claims there is a connection between genetic knowledge and well-being. The two views are, at a high level of generality, making the same claim. I want to start, then, by highlighting the essential features of the Profound Prudential Good view so that I can be clear about how the Significant Interest view is different.

The Profound Prudential Good view maintains that genetic knowledge has *non-optional, near universal, weighty* importance for well-being.[6] What does this mean? Genetic knowledge is *non-optional* (according to this view) in a metaphysically weak sense: as a matter of fact, given the world we live in and the kinds of creatures we are, acquiring genetic knowledge is a prudential

---

[5] And usually decisive. A reminder that showing that it is usually decisive is the work of chapter 6.

[6] I've coined the name for the view. The most sustained philosophical articulation of the view comes from David Velleman, although his notion of "genetic knowledge" is considerably more demanding than the one I am using here. Velleman thinks of genetic knowledge in terms of being substantially acquainted with (indeed, ideally raised by) one's genetic parents. Velleman would also resist my assimilation of his account of the importance of genetic knowledge to a concern about well-being as opposed to respect. I say a little more about this feature of this view presently. See J. David Velleman, "The Gift of Life," *Philosophy & Public Affairs* 36, no. 3 (2008): 245–66; J. David Velleman, "Family History," *Philosophical Papers* 34, no. 3 (2005): 357–78. Another example of this kind of view comes from Tom Frame who—like Velleman—emphasizes the importance of children "living with both their [genetic] parents as the foremost foundation from which they can understand themselves and their place in the world." Thomas R. Frame, *Children on Demand: The Ethics of Defying Nature* (Sydney: UNSW Press, 2008), 55. Velleman's arguments are trenchantly criticized by Sally Haslanger, "Family, Ancestry, and Self," in *Resisting Reality: Social Construction and Social Critique* (New York: Oxford University Press, 2012), 158–182. The difference between my conception of genetic knowledge and Velleman's doesn't matter for my purpose here, which is just to pull out the formal features of the view according to which genetic knowledge—on *some* plausible interpretation of what it is—is a profound prudential good. A direct argument against the Profound Prudential Good view—including the version with Velleman's demanding sense of "genetic knowledge"—is offered in chapter 4.

good that cannot be replaced by some other prudential good without significant loss. Implicit in this idea is that having genetic knowledge is important for basically everyone: it has *universal* importance. Perhaps it is not transparent to everyone that it prudentially matters—they might not think explicitly in terms of the prudential value of having genetic knowledge—but its universal importance can be seen in a vast array of cultural products and practices that emphasize the importance of knowing who your genetic parents are.[7] Finally, something might have non-optional, universal prudential importance . . . but not much. The Profound Prudential Good view, unsurprisingly, maintains that genetic knowledge is not one of those things: it is a very weighty prudential good. According to this view, someone who lacks genetic knowledge is missing something that matters a lot.

These three features of the view—non-optionality, universality, and significant weight—come through in the idea that genetic knowledge is all but required for the kind of self-knowledge that is central to healthy identity formation. I say a lot more about what this means in the next chapter, but the basic thought is simple enough. Someone who lacks genetic knowledge is missing a central source of self-knowledge that allows a person to make sense of themselves as the kind of person they are and the kind of person they could be. As David Velleman puts it:

> When adoptees go in search of their biological parents and siblings, there is a literal sense in which they are searching for themselves. They are searching for the closest thing to a mirror in which to catch an external and candid view of what they are like in more than mere appearance. Not knowing any biological relatives must be like wandering in a world without reflective surfaces, permanently self-blind.
>
> Children denied a knowledge of only one biological parent are not entirely cut off from this view of themselves, but they are cut off from one half of it. Their estrangement even from one parent, or half-brothers and -sisters, must still be a deprivation, because it estranges them from people who would be familiar without any prior acquaintance, people with whom they would enjoy that natural familiarity which would be so revealing about themselves.[8]

---

[7] For some examples, see Velleman, "Family History," 369.

[8] Velleman, "Family History," 368. Although he does not use the term, Velleman's view is a version of the idea that people who do not know their genetic progenitors experience so-called "genetic bewilderment." For discussion of how the concept of genetic bewilderment is deployed in scholarship on both adoption and gamete donation, see Kimberly Leighton, "Addressing the Harms

If Velleman is right about this and genetic knowledge has non-optional, universal, weighty prudential value, then there is a tight connection between having genetic knowledge and well-being. From there, it is easy to see the outline of an argument for why intended parents have a weighty, and probably decisive, reason to use an open donor: in conceiving a child with anonymously donated gametes, intended parents effectively deprive their child of a weighty prudential good.

Crucially, proponents of the Profound Prudential Good view need not claim that people who lack genetic knowledge do not have lives worth living or even flourishing lives. The claim, rather, is just that a life without genetic knowledge is substantially disadvantaged or, to use Velleman's term, "truncated" even if, overall, the person's life goes quite well (and the person living it is very pleased to exist).[9]

But now one might wonder: If lives that lack genetic knowledge are (well) worth living, what objection could there be to creating such lives? Indeed, why not say that a child who is created without access to genetic knowledge has nothing to complain about since their life is good enough *and* lacking genetic knowledge was a condition of their existence (since if the parents had used an open donor, *this* child wouldn't have come into existence)? Velleman's answer is that the threshold for permissibly creating a life is considerably higher than the threshold for that life being one worth *continuing*.[10] In other words, a human life that lacks X might be (well) worth continuing, but intentionally creating a human life that will lack X is impermissible. The basic thought behind this claim is that personhood has a value that demands respect and, in order to respect that value, "we are obligated, in creating human lives, to create ones in which that value is more likely to flower and least likely to be disfigured."[11] So if you're going to bring someone

---

of Not Knowing One's Heredity: Lessons from Genealogical Bewilderment," *Adoption & Culture* 3 (2012): 64. Leighton argues that appeals to genealogical bewilderment as an independent phenomenon are ill-grounded and that, instead, the harm scholars take themselves to be merely describing is in fact *generated* by the claim that people need to know their genetic progenitors for healthy-identity formation. I say more about this in chapter 5.

[9] Velleman, "The Gift of Life," 255.

[10] J. David Velleman, "III. Love and Nonexistence," *Philosophy & Public Affairs* 36, no. 3 (2008): 273–74.

[11] Velleman, "The Gift of Life," 254. A detailed account of Velleman's argument and how it relates to the purported prudential badness of lacking genetic knowledge can be found in Olivia Schuman, "The Value of Genetic Ties as Ethical Justification for Banning Gamete Donor Anonymity," PhD dissertation, York University, 2020, https://yorkspace.library.yorku.ca/xmlui/handle/10315/37789. I am indebted to Schuman's work in helping me think through these issues.

into existence, you best ensure that their life will not lack for goods that will disfigure the person's life if they are missing, even if a life without those goods is well worth continuing. If you think, as Velleman does, that having genetic knowledge is a good of this kind—because of its connection to forming one's identity—then intentionally creating someone who will lack it will not clear the bar for permissible procreation.[12]

My goal here is not to argue against the Profound Prudential Good view, but simply to highlight its defining elements so as to differentiate it from the Significant Interest view. But I think it is important to briefly note that findings on donor-conceived children and their families do not obviously support the idea that people who lack genetic knowledge are missing a profound prudential good or living "disfigured" lives. To put it simply, the research on donor-conceived children and their families suggests that the kids (and their families) are alright: the families function well and the children do just fine.[13] Moreover, among donor-conceived people who know they are donor-conceived, the desire to find one's genetic progenitor is not universal.[14] This is not what you would expect if donor-conceived people were deprived of a profound prudential good, even granting that one's life can be well worth living without it.

These findings are consistent with the Profound Prudential Good view. Those who are not bothered by their lack of genetic knowledge could just be

---

[12] So proponents of this view can admit that once someone exists, it may be best for that person—and fully compatible with respecting them—to put them up for adoption. Velleman, "The Gift of Life," 252.

[13] And to the extent that there are findings to the contrary, this is usually because there are serious confounding factors at play such as (for example) the fact that the parents didn't tell the child she was donor-conceived until well into the child's life. For a great overview of the social science, see Susan Golombok, *Modern Families: Parents and Children in New Family Forms* (Cambridge, UK: Cambridge University Press, 2015), chapter 4.

[14] A 2009 study found that 34% of donor-conceived people who knew about their status as donor-conceived people (almost always *via* parental disclosure) describe themselves as currently "indifferent" to that information. See Vasanti Jadva et al., "The Experiences of Adolescents and Adults Conceived by Sperm Donation: Comparisons by Age of Disclosure and Family Type," *Human Reproduction* 24, no. 8 (2009): 1909–19. In a 2003 study of donor-conceived people being raised in lesbian households (all the kids were between 7 and 17 years old), over 50% said they did not want any information about their donor. However, it is important to note that when asked why, some of these children cited concerns about hurting their social mother(s). Others, however, simply expressed no interest on their own behalf. See Katrien Vanfraussen, Ingrid Ponjaert-Kristoffersen, and Anne Brewaeys, "Why Do Children Want to Know More about the Donor? The Experience of Youngsters Raised in Lesbian Families," *Journal of Psychosomatic Obstetrics & Gynecology* 24, no. 1 (2003): 31–38. Beeson et al. found that 82% of donor-conceived people who knew they were donor-conceived expressed an interest to "be in contact some day with their donor." Diane R. Beeson, Patricia K. Jennings, and Wendy Kramer, "Offspring Searching for Their Sperm Donors: How Family Type Shapes the Process," *Human Reproduction* 26, no. 9 (2011): 2419. I will come back to these statistics below (p. 67).

wrong about what matters. More plausibly, you might think that the studies in question, while demonstrating that donor-conceived people do well enough, don't capture the ways in which their flourishing is negatively impacted by a lack of genetic knowledge. That is, you might think that the studies have not, in effect, operationalized the disadvantage of lacking genetic knowledge.[15] Or you might claim that the fact that very many donor-conceived people *do* seek out genetic knowledge is strong evidence that there is something very important missing from their lives.

The upshot is that I don't pretend to have settled the matter here. My full response to the Profound Prudential Good view comes in the next chapter. For now, my point is just that the sociology on donor-conceived people and their families gives us reason to wonder whether the Profound Prudential Good view oversells the prudential import of genetic knowledge. Assuming for now that it does, the question is this: Is there another argument based on well-being for using an open donor?

2. Well-being and significant interests

There is! Let's start with this thought about well-being:

> **Well-being and significant interests:** How well your life goes for you is partly (if not largely) a function of how successful you are in satisfying your non-instrumental significant, worthwhile interests. If you satisfy a non-instrumental, significant worthwhile interest then—to that extent—your life goes better for you.

I'll call this the Well-Being Principle. By a *significant* interest, I mean an interest that matters quite a lot to the person who has it. I enjoy peeling labels off beer bottles in bars. Other things being equal, I will choose a beer bottle with a label so that I can peel the label off. Peeling-labels-off-beer-bottles-in-bars is an interest of mine. It is not a significant interest.

I offer no theory of what makes an interest significant except to say (1) significance is scalar: one interest can be more significant than another and less significant than still another; and (2) the significance of an interest is partly a

---

[15] This suggestion was made by David Velleman at a conference at NYU on the ethics of gamete donation and echoed by a number of donor-conceived people in the room.

matter of the space, so to speak, it takes up in a person's mental economy (do they think about it a lot?) and the extent to which they organize their lives around it. Significant interests play a structuring role in a person's life and self-conception.

But not all significant interests are covered by the Well-Being Principle. Pretty much everyone has a significant interest in getting enough sleep. But such an interest is normally merely instrumental, which is to say that people are interested in it only for something else it allows them to do (like: making it through the day without feeling awful, being able to do better work, enjoying the company of those around them). Consider, by way of contrast, the interest that most people have in fostering a meaningful relationship with their children or the interest that most nurses have in providing care for their patients. Though fulfilling these interests might well lead to parents and nurses getting something—such as a paycheck in the case of a nurse—the interest is not *just* about getting something else. Instead, fulfilling the interest (fostering the relationship with your kids, caring for your patients) is valued directly. That is what I mean when I say that the interests are "non-instrumental."

This doesn't mean that fulfilling the interest has no instrumental value; the fact that nurses get paid makes that clear. It also doesn't mean that the interest is not valued as a part of some broader interest the person has. Perhaps the nurse has a broader interest in helping others. Nursing is *how* he helps others. His interest in nursing, we might say, is the specification of his broader interest in helping others, which must be done by doing something more specific (nursing, running a non-profit, teaching). The point here is that while we can often tell a story about how a person's significant interests serve some broader goal a person has, that doesn't mean that the interest is merely an *instrument* for bringing about the broader goal. It is, rather, the embodiment or instantiation of the broader goal. In short: non-instrumental significant interests can be valued by people as *part* of a broader goal or interest.

Let's make explicit something that has only been implicit to this point: when I talk about a person "having an interest" I have in mind a *subjective* interest (i.e. something that a person actually wants to satisfy) and not an *objective* interest (i.e. something that it is in the person's interest to have satisfied whether they actually want to satisfy it or not). In light of this clarification, the Well-Being Principle might now strike some as highly suspect. Why think that satisfying a person's significant interests is good for them?

Notice, though, that the Well-Being Principle does not say that satisfying *whatever* non-instrumental significant interests a person has is good for them. Rather, it restricts the relevant class of interests to those that are *worth-while*. I explained above what I mean by calling an interest "worthwhile": it is neither trivial nor morally problematic. What it means for an interest to be trivial or morally problematic is none too clear. I don't offer a general account of these terms. But I do discuss why the interest in genetic knowledge is neither trivial nor morally problematic.[16] For now, the point is that by including the "worthwhile" qualification, I hope to make palatable the idea that a person's life goes better to the extent they satisfy their significant interests, even when we understand those interests as subjective interests.

The Well-Being Principle is, I think, intuitively attractive. Think about your own non-instrumental, significant interests (from here on out, I'm going to drop the "non-instrumental" for ease of exposition). To the extent that you have been able to satisfy them—and satisfying them might be an ongoing activity owing to the nature of the interest—then you will, I suspect, think your life has gone better because of it. If your attempts to satisfy have been frustrated, you will feel, well, *frustrated*: "Here is something that has not gone well, or as well as it could have, in my life," you might say. "I have not succeeded when it comes to this thing that matters to me." From a first-person perspective, satisfaction of interests seems central to one's own flourishing.

Moreover, as outsiders we will surely endorse that first-person assessment if we think your significant interests are worthwhile, i.e. are non-trivial and not morally problematic. Indeed, to the extent that a person's significant interests are worthwhile, they are plausibly a substantial source of what gives their life meaning.[17] Some will think that satisfaction of a person's significant interests contributes to their well-being *only if* the interests are worthwhile.[18] But we need not take a stand on that contentious claim here, since the Well-Being Principle makes a weaker claim: *if* your significant interests are worthwhile, then satisfying them makes your life go better. This is a very intuitive

---

[16] Briefly below and then in detail in chapters 4 and 5.

[17] The Well-Being Principle, which weds subjective interest to something like "objective worthwhileness," takes its inspiration from Susan Wolf's conception of meaning according to which, "meaning arises when subjective attraction meets objective attractiveness." Susan Wolf, *Meaning in Life and Why It Matters*, (Princeton, NJ: Princeton University Press, 2012), 9. Having said that, I think the principle could easily be taken on by those that ascribe to preference- or desire-based theories of well-being since it partially articulates the heart of their views. According to these views (roughly) what makes something good for you is that it satisfies some non-instrumental interest (desire, preference) of yours. So satisfying your non-instrumental, worthwhile interests will make your life go better for you.

[18] This is what I think. I think it's what I think, anyhow. I'm perennially in a muddle on this issue.

thought, whatever you think about the connection between the satisfaction of someone's non-worthwhile significant interests and their well-being.

With the Well-Being Principle in hand, we are in a position to forge an initial connection between having genetic knowledge and well-being:

1. If someone satisfies a significant, worthwhile interest, then, to that extent, their life goes better for them.
2. There are some people for whom having genetic knowledge is a significant, worthwhile interest.
3. So, if those people have genetic knowledge, then their lives go better for them (to that extent).

This argument for a connection between genetic knowledge and increased well-being posits no special connection between genetic knowledge and well-being. Rather the connection falls out of a more general, very simple story about how well-being is connected to satisfying significant, worthwhile interests *whatever they may be*. To see this, notice that we could run the argument for an entirely different significant, worthwhile interest some people have:

1. If someone satisfies a significant, worthwhile interest, then, to that extent, their life goes better for them.
2. There are some people for whom competing to build cars with the loudest possible stereo—which is known as "dB drag-racing"[19]—is a worthwhile significant interest.
3. So, if those people compete to build cars with the loudest possible stereo, then their lives go better for them (to that extent).

At this point, you might feel let down. If all I mean by asserting a connection between having genetic knowledge and well-being is that there are *some* people for whom acquiring genetic knowledge is prudentially good—in virtue of those particular people having a worthwhile significant interest in genetic knowledge—then there is nothing to object to. I have not shown that there is anything resembling a *deep* connection between genetic knowledge and well-being. Indeed, for all I have said, I could just as easily have written

[19] See *This American Life*, "Crunk in the Trunk," December 12, 2017, https://www.thisamericanlife.org/279/auto-show/act-one.

this chapter (or a whole book!) about the connection between well-being and dB drag-racing or any other idiosyncratic worthwhile interest.

An interest in dB drag-racing is a *very* idiosyncratic significant interest. Other examples of such interests might include dog breeding, stamp collecting, visiting every Major League Baseball stadium, being a practicing Jew, or being a foster parent. But not all the interests are idiosyncratic. Some are (very nearly) universal. Following (and slightly modifying) Rawls, I will call these *primary interests*.[20] Primary interests are interests that everyone can be presumed to have no matter what other interests they have.[21] Primary interests are always significant interests.

If genetic knowledge were a worthwhile primary interest, then there would be a fairly deep connection between having genetic knowledge and well-being: we would have identified a (near) universal ingredient of well-being. I have, however, already ruled out pursuing this argumentative route. But now it looks like I have a problem. For if the interest in genetic knowledge is merely idiosyncratic, then it seems I am stuck with the very weak conclusion that an interest in genetic knowledge is related to well-being in much the same way an interest in dB drag-racing is.

But that is not right. To see why, consider what follows from the fact that an interest is a primary interest: it is foreseeable that any given person has it. The same is typically not true of idiosyncratic interests. It is not at all foreseeable that anyone you happen to meet has a significant interest in dB drag-racing. Indeed, that interest is *so* idiosyncratic that it would be irrational to predict that any given person has it. In general, then, the fact that an interest is idiosyncratic makes it irrational to predict that any given person has it and especially irrational to predict that any given young child will *come* to have it.

The idiosyncratic interest in having genetic knowledge, however, is an exception. It is an idiosyncratic interest where, with just one bit of information, it is rational to predict not just that someone has it but also that someone will come to have it. That information is that the person is donor-conceived. What makes the prediction rational is that it is very common, though not universal, among donor-conceived people to be significantly interested in acquiring genetic knowledge.[22]

[20] John Rawls, *Justice as Fairness: A Restatement* (Cambridge, MA: Harvard University Press, 2001), 58–59.

[21] Neil Levy, "Forced to Be Free? Increasing Patient Autonomy by Constraining It," *Journal of Medical Ethics* 40, no. 5 (2014): 294.

[22] If what I said at the end of chapter 1 is right, then the interest in genetic knowledge is probably common among the population at large though rarely foregrounded in people's minds because they

In support of this claim, consider the following four pieces of evidence. First, there is burgeoning interest in online forums and registries for donor-conceived people. The Donor Sibling Registry, which Rhonda E. Harris and Laura Shanner describe as the "most important, non-governmental, voluntary registry and matching service in the world,"[23] was created in 2000. In 2005, "The DSR reported 4,000 families registered [. . .]; in 2006, over 7000 [. . .]; in 2009, 24,000 registrants [. . .]; in July 2011, 31,248 registrants [. . .]; by November 2012 . . . over, 38,300 registrants."[24]

Second, in a 2003, researchers did a study with parents who conceived with an open donor and had either disclosed or planned to disclose this fact to their adolescent child. The researchers asked the parents what they thought their child's reaction would be to learning they were donor-conceived and that they could learn the identity of their donor. The researchers report that:

Many [parents] already knew how the child felt. Most parents expected or knew that their child felt at least neutral, if not moderately positive, about the donor. Among the few parents who anticipated negative feelings, it was when the child had not yet been told about his or her donor conception. Some thought their child would have concerns and/or be anxious about the donor, such as what he would be like and whether he would be willing to meet him or her and like him or her, nevertheless similar numbers also reported that their child looked forward to possible meetings. *Most of all, however, the overwhelming response from the children was curiosity about the donor.*[25]

Third, in a 2009 study of donor-conceived people whose status was disclosed to them, only 21% described themselves as currently "indifferent." The

---

already take the interest to be met. If that's right, then the interest is not idiosyncratic but really very common. The argument would still go through since all I need is that it is foreseeable that any given person is likely to be interested in having genetic knowledge.

[23] R. Harris and L. Shanner, "Seeking Answers in the Ether: Longing to Know One's Origins Is Evident from Donor Conception Websites," in *The Right to Know One's Origins: Assisted Human Reproduction and the Best Interests of Children*, ed. Juliet Ruth Guichon, Ian Mitchell, and Michelle Giroux (Brussels: ASP, 2012), 61.

[24] Although, according to John Appleby (personal correspondence), many of the people who have signed up for the DSR are *parents* of donor-conceived children, and not the donor-conceived people themselves. See Tabitha Freeman et al., "Gamete Donation: Parents' Experiences of Searching for Their Child's Donor Siblings and Donor," *Human Reproduction* 24, no. 3 (2009): 505–16.

[25] Joanna E. Scheib, Maura Riordan, and Susan Rubin, "Choosing Identity-Release Sperm Donors: The Parents' Perspective 13–18 Years Later," *Human Reproduction* 18, no. 5 (2003): 1124.

majority (69%) described themselves as curious.[26] Fourth, and finally, in a 2014 study, 82% of donor-conceived people who knew they were donor-conceived expressed an interest to "be in contact someday with their donor."[27]

Now we need to be cautious with these kinds of findings. Participants in both the 2009 and 2014 studies I just cited were recruited via the Donor Sibling Registry. It is no surprise to learn that people who have registered for the DSR have *some* interest in acquiring genetic knowledge. If they didn't—if they were entirely uninterested in acquiring genetic knowledge—they probably wouldn't have signed up for the DSR in the first place (though it's possible their parents got the ball rolling).[28] More generally, donor-conceived people who are genuinely uninterested in acquiring genetic knowledge are less likely to participate in these kinds of studies, partly because they are less likely to learn about these studies in the first place and to participate in them when they do.

Even so, the four bits of evidence above taken together suggest that having genetic knowledge is a very common interest among donor-conceived people, even if it is not universal. It looks like a good, though by no means certain, bet that any given donor-conceived person either has or will develop a significant interest in having genetic knowledge. It is different in that respect from idiosyncratic interests like stamp collecting, dog breeding, or dB drag-racing. Other things being equal, it is not a good bet that someone is interested in them. And, if they are young children, it is not a good bet that they *will* be interested in those things.[29] These idiosyncratic interests are not *foreseeable* interests. The interest in genetic knowledge, on the other hand, is foreseeable, at least for donor-conceived people. Moreover, it is worthwhile in the minimal sense I intend: it is neither trivial nor morally problematic.[30]

In light of this, what can we say about the connection between satisfying an interest in genetic knowledge and the well-being of donor-conceived people? In general, donor-conceived people are significantly interested in genetic knowledge. And, as the Well-Being Principle tells us, satisfying

---

[26] Jadva et al., "The Experiences of Adolescents and Adults Conceived by Sperm Donation," 1913.

[27] Beeson, Jennings, and Kramer, "Offspring Searching for Their Sperm Donors," 2419.

[28] Indeed, in light of this observation, it is striking that as much as 21% of respondents in the 2009 study described themselves as currently "indifferent." Thank you to an anonymous reviewer for emphasizing these concerns about selection bias.

[29] Parents play a huge role in shaping what interests a child will have. So perhaps they are in a position to make different bets than a stranger about what interests their child will develop. I consider this possibility below (pp. 75–78).

[30] I have not argued for this yet. I address it briefly below and then in depth in chapters 4 and 5 (pp. 78–80).

one's worthwhile significant interests contributes to one's well-being. There is, then, a general connection between donor-conceived people's improved well-being and their having genetic knowledge.

This connection is not as tight as it would be if the interest in genetic knowledge were (near) universal: then there would a connection between (almost) everyone's well-being and having genetic knowledge. Moreover, the connection I have argued for is not as deep as it would be if genetic knowledge had non-optional, weighty prudential importance: then we would be able to bypass the empirical point about people's subjective interest in it and just point to the prudential importance of having genetic knowledge. In other words, the account I have offered of the connection between having genetic knowledge and well-being is somewhat weak.

However, it is strong enough in the following sense: it is enough to ground the argument that intended parents have a weighty reason to conceive with an open donor. And this "strong enough" approach is precisely what I am going for. We don't need to defend the (implausible, in my view) claim that having genetic knowledge is profoundly prudentially important in order to show that intended parents have a weighty reason to conceive with an open donor. As we will see, it is enough that, as a matter of fact, an interest in genetic knowledge is a worthwhile, foreseeable interest, at least for donor-conceived people.

3. Parents and their children's future significant interests

How do we get from the idea that acquiring genetic knowledge is a worthwhile, foreseeable interest of many donor-conceived people to the conclusion that parents have a weighty reason to use an open donor? It starts with a very basic assumption: parents have a weighty obligation to promote their children's overall well-being. Some version of this assumption is undeniable. Even so, it is not entirely clear what it amounts to, since it tells us nothing about *when* parents have the obligation and what, exactly, its object is, i.e. well-being *at a time* or *across a life*? To see this, consider how we might unpack the assumption:

Parents have a weighty obligation [**at all times of their child's life**//**only when their child is young**] to promote the child's overall well-being [**across their child's life**//**only when their child is young**].

Rather than walking through all the possibilities, we can help ourselves to an uncontroversial specification of the assumption:

> Parents have a weighty obligation **at least when their child is young** to promote the child's overall well-being **across their child's life.**

A key responsibility of parents is to prepare their children for adult life. A parent who is focused on their child's well-being only when the child is young plausibly should accede to all, or at least most, requests for more ice cream. A total lack of concern for developing traits, habits, and skills that will serve the child well in the future would be perfectly appropriate if the child does not have a future past childhood. But assuming that they do, a central responsibility of parents is to make decisions *now* for the sake of their child's well-being as an adult.

Actually meeting this obligation is one of the central challenges of parenthood. But the Well-Being Principle gives us some guidance for how parents can go about meeting it. Suppose, for example, that I *know* my child will develop a significant interest in dB drag-racing no matter what I do. The Well-Being Principle tells me that, other things being equal, satisfying this interest will make my child's life better. Now, we could imagine a scenario where I reasonably believe that, all things considered, satisfying this interest will make her life worse—perhaps we live in a society where dB drag-racers are severely persecuted. But suppose it is not reasonable for me to believe that satisfying my child's future interest will make her life worse. Then the Well-Being Principle, combined with the assumption that I have a weighty obligation when my child is young to promote her well-being across her life, tells me that I have a weighty reason to prepare the ground for my child to succeed in satisfying this significant interest (by, perhaps, signing her up for engineering camps or taking her to dB drag-races).

More generally, parents' obligation to promote their children's well-being, when combined with the Well-Being Principle, implies that parents have a weighty reason to prepare the ground for their children to satisfy their worthwhile, future significant interests unless the parents reasonably believe doing so will make their child less well-off overall. I'll call this the Future Significant Interests Principle.

How should parents go about acting on the Future Significant Interests Principle? The example I just offered might suggest that the principle is practically idle: parents cannot know, with any degree of confidence, that their child will develop a significant interest in dB drag-racing. More generally, parents are largely in the dark with respect to what their child's future significant interests will be. In fact, one of the great sources of joy and anxiety in parenting is wondering about, and watching, what kind of person your child will become, what will move and motivate them, what pursuits and passions will shape their life.

But it is easy to overstate the uncertainty parents face about their child's future significant interests. For, as we saw above, there are different kinds of future significant interests. Some are foreseeable, while others are not. It is highly foreseeable that a child will have interests that are in the set of primary interests. And there are other interests that, while not universal, are sufficiently common that it is foreseeable that a child will likely develop them as well. Raising a family might be an example. It is not a (near) universal interest, but it is a good bet that a child will develop this interest. And then there are interests that, while not common among the general population, are nonetheless foreseeable given the circumstances. These are idiosyncratic foreseeable interests. The interest in having genetic knowledge among donor-conceived people is an example of such an interest.[31] So, for intended parents of donor-conceived children, it is foreseeable that their child will likely develop a significant interest in having genetic knowledge.

The Future Significant Interests Principle, then, isn't a true-but-practically-idle principle. Parents *do* have a good idea about what some of their children's future significant interests will be. And when it comes to at least some of those interests, parents can prepare the ground for their children to satisfy those interests. The Future Significant Interests Principle tells parents that they have a weighty reason to do so (unless they reasonably think doing so will be deleterious to their child's overall well-being). The upshot is that if having genetic knowledge is a significant, foreseeable interest for donor-conceived people, then parents of donor-conceived children have a weighty reason—when the child is young—to prepare the ground for their child to satisfy that interest (unless they reasonably think doing so will be deleterious to their child's overall well-being).

What does this have to do with whether or not *intended parents* have a weighty reason to use an open donor? After all, when that decision is being made there is, as yet, no child to whom one is obligated. How could the

---

[31] Although if what I said above is correct, then it is an example of a very common, though not universal, interest. Either way, my argument goes through (p. 68).

Future Significant Interests Principle apply to intended parents? The answer is that intended parents will be obligated to their future child, *whoever it will be*, in the way described by the Future Significant Interests Principle. In planning to conceive a child, intended parents knowingly and voluntarily take on a role which is partly defined in terms of having a weighty obligation to promote the well-being of their future child. The obligation articulated in the Future Significant Interests Principle is in the offing. And this obligates intended parents to take steps *now* to put themselves in the position to meet that coming obligation.[32] So, if they will have a weighty reason to help their child—whoever it is—satisfy a foreseeable, future significant interest in having genetic knowledge, then they have a weighty reason to decide *now* to use an open donor. Doing so will enable them, when their child exists, to meet their parental obligations.

4. Objections

The Significant Interest view maintains that intended parents have a weighty reason to use an open donor in virtue of (a) the foreseeability that donor-conceived people will likely develop a significant, worthwhile interest in having genetic knowledge; (b) the connection between satisfying one's significant, worthwhile interests and one's well-being; and (c) parents' obligation to promote their children's well-being. Now, someone might agree with all that, but deny that intended parents have a *decisive* reason to use an open donor. I return to this claim in chapter 6. Right now, I want to consider two objections to the conclusion that the Significant Interest view has even identified a weighty reason to use an open donor.

---

[32] It is true that in deciding to act so as to put themselves in a good position to help the future child satisfy their (the child's) foreseeable interest, the parents are making a decision about *which* child will come to exist (since they are choosing between different donated gametes). But that doesn't matter. For the parents are, in effect, making a choice between bringing into existence (a) a child where they (the parents) are knowingly likely to fail in some way with respect to their obligation to help promote the child's well-being and (b) a child where they are in an excellent position to meet their obligation to help promote the child's well-being. I say more about this in chapter 1 when I discuss the non-identity problem, but my assumption here is that intended parents have a weighty reason to choose to bring the second child into existence rather than the first.

4.1. First objection: more harm than good?

I have claimed that intended parents have a weighty reason to use an open donor *unless they reasonably think doing so will be deleterious to the child's overall well-being.* A critic might claim that it *is,* in general, reasonable to think that using an open donor will be overall deleterious to the child's well-being. Perhaps coming to know the identity of your donor is likely to cause emotional distress, or a severe disruption in your sense of self, or on-going familial disputes. Maybe, as a result, donor-conceived people are, in general, better off not knowing who their donor is in the first place. If some version of this is right, then generally speaking intended parents don't have a weighty reason to use an open donor (at least as far as my argument is concerned).

This objection puts the burden of proof squarely on the objector to explain whether, in fact, parents could reasonably believe that aiming to satisfy the (likely, future) significant interest in having genetic knowledge *through use of an open donor* will be overall deleterious to their child's well-being. The bit in italics is important. It is not hard to see how satisfying a person's interest in having genetic knowledge by helping them to track down an *anonymous* donor might not go well for the donor-conceived person. Anonymous donors are sometimes happy to be identified, but sometimes they are not. As Freeman et al. explain, "Contact experiences may lead to disappointment, bitterness and distress, particularly if the expectations of those involved are incompatible."[33] They share one donor-conceived adult's account of a negative experience:

> Although [my donor] is glad that I was born, he is not proud to have participated in donor conception . . . It is a pretty bad feeling that my life has been such a source of shame and embarrassment, through no fault of my own, by the people who brought me into this world.[34]

Overall, however, the evidence we have about contact between donor-conceived people and their donors suggests that it is usually, though not

---

[33] Tabitha Freeman, John B. Appleby, and Vasanti Jadva, "Identifiable Donors and Siblings," in *Reproductive Donation,* ed. Martin Richards, Guido Pennings, and John Appleby (Cambridge: Cambridge University Press, 2012), 260.

[34] Freeman, Appleby, and Jadva, "Identifiable Donors and Siblings," 260–61.

universally, a positive experience. Freemen et al. report the following on a public program in Victoria, Australia, to "operationalize the complex process of linking donor relations": "So far, there have been few reports of negative outcomes of contact involving donors or half-siblings, with those who meet tending to get on well and stay in touch."[35] More generally, Freeman et al. note that studies about donor contact involving "face-to-face" meetings were positive:

> Most meetings between sperm donor offspring and their donor were found to be mutually beneficial. The large majority noticed and enjoyed perceived similarities, particularly in terms of physical appearance, which in some cases contributed to a sense of connectedness. Prior anxieties were frequently allayed by meeting in person, and the reality of the meeting could exceed anticipations and be an emotional "bonding" encounter for all.[36]

A 2010 study by Jadva et al. found that 70% of donor-conceived people who made contact with their donor had a "very positive experience," while none had a "very negative experience."[37]

It is reasonable to assume that if contact between donor-conceived people and their previously anonymous donors is very often positive, the same will be true of contact between donor-conceived people and donors who agreed in advance to make their identities available. Of course, people can change their minds and, even if they don't, contact might not go well. But on the whole, it is safe to assume that open donors are willing (in some cases perhaps waiting) for their genetic offspring to get in touch. Barring special circumstances, then, it does not seem reasonable for intended parents to believe that putting their child in a position to have genetic knowledge by using an open donor will be overall deleterious to the child's well-being.

[35] Freeman, Appleby, and Jadva, "Identifiable Donors and Siblings," 286.

[36] Freeman, Appleby, and Jadva, "Identifiable Donors and Siblings," 285. They note, however, that there have been "very few" studies of this kind and that "first meetings are just one stage in the complex process of forming connections."

[37] Vasanti Jadva et al., "Experiences of Offspring Searching for and Contacting Their Donor Siblings and Donor," *Reproductive Biomedicine Online* 20, no. 4 (2010): 530. Of the remaining 30%, 10% had a "fairly positive" experience, 10% had a "neutral" experience, and 10% had a "fairly negative" experience." It is worth noting that the sample size (n = 10) was very small.

4.2. Second objection: parental influence and foreseeable interests

I have claimed that a donor-conceived person's interest in genetic knowledge is foreseeable. One might think this is true in one sense: for any given donor-conceived person, it is a good bet they will develop a significant interest in having genetic knowledge. The implicit claim is that because the interest is foreseeable in this sense, parents of donor-conceived children should assume that *their* child is very likely to have an interest in genetic knowledge. But surely this paints the wrong picture of the relationship between parents, their children, and their children's interests. I have, in effect, been imagining parents asking themselves, "What will my child's future significant interests be?," as though this is purely an epistemic question. Talk of the interest being "foreseeable" encourages this reading. It suggests that what a child's future significant interests will be is independent of the answers the parents come up with. Asking, "What will my child's future significant interests be?" is, according to this picture, like asking, "What will the weather be tomorrow?" How I answer the question plays no role in determining the actual answer.

But parents play a huge role in determining what significant interests their children will have. And this means that while some interests might be very common indeed, that doesn't necessarily give parents good reasons to think *their* child will develop such interests. Consider, for example, what is surely a foreseeable future interest of most children in the United States: being involved in a religious community. But children of parents in the United States who practice no religion are very likely to *not* have any significant interest in religion precisely because their parents had no such interest.[38] To the extent that parents know this—and indeed intentionally inculcate a lack of interest in religion—they have no reason to do anything when their child is young to help their child satisfy an interest in religious practice. This is because their child is very unlikely to develop this interest even though, in general, it is foreseeable that any given child in the United States will likely develop the interest. The same might be true when it comes to the interest in genetic knowledge. If parents emphasize that having genetic knowledge is thoroughly unimportant, then, perhaps, it is very likely that their child will believe it is unimportant and so develop no significant interest in having it. The parents,

---

[38] Vern L. Bengtson, Susan Harris, and Norella M. Putney, *Families and Faith: How Religion Is Passed Down across Generations* (New York: Oxford University Press, 2017), 152.

then, would have no reason to prepare the ground for the child to acquire genetic knowledge and, so, no reason to use an open donor (at least so far as the Significant Interest view is concerned). I call this the Parental Influence objection.

One response to the objection is to claim that to the best of their abilities, parents should not influence a child's future significant interests. Whatever significant interests a child develops as she matures into adulthood should be, in some sense, up to her. In other words, parents should keep their children's future as open as possible. As a result, it would be a wrongful imposition of the child's future autonomy to actively inculcate in the child a lack of interest in genetic knowledge.[39]

This response to the Parental Influence objection is open to critique on at least two fronts. The first is practical: parents' influence over their children's value and interests is simply unavoidable. Indeed, attempting to *avoid* it really is just another way of shaping future values and interests.[40] The second critique is moral: even if shaping is, to some extent, avoidable (and surely to some extent it is), parents are entitled to shape at least some of their child's interests and values in some ways. As Brighouse and Swift have argued, some distinctive goods—for both children and parents—can only be realized in the context of intimate family bonds. And part of the way those bonds are created is by parents sharing their interests and values with their children.[41]

Perhaps defenders of the open future approach have compelling responses to these critiques.[42] I want to present what I think is a more fruitful response to the Parental Influence objection. It begins by granting the painfully obvious point that parents play a huge role in shaping the future significant

---

[39] This is a version of Feinberg's well-known view that children have a right to an "open future." Joel Feinberg, "The Child's Right to an Open Future," in *Justice, Politics, and the Family* (New York: Routledge, 2015), 145–60. Matthew Clayton defends what he calls "parental anti-perfectionism," according to which "it is not a legitimate aim for those responsible for raising a child to enroll her into particular comprehensive practices." By "comprehensive practices" Clayton has in mind practices that revolve around, for example, "particular religious goals, occupational aims, and conceptions of the kinds of family and sexuality that are worthy of pursuit." Matthew Clayton, "Anti-Perfectionist Childrearing," in *The Nature of Children's Well-Being* (New York: Springer, 2015), 126, 130. See also Matthew Clayton, *Justice and Legitimacy in Upbringing* (Oxford University Press, 2006).

[40] Claudia Mills, "The Child's Right to an Open Future?," *Journal of Social Philosophy* 34, no. 4 (2003): 499–509. She also makes a series of other criticisms of the Open Future Argument.

[41] Harry Brighouse and Adam Swift, *Family Values: The Ethics of Parent-Child Relationships* (Princeton, NJ: Princeton University Press, 2014), 153–61. As Brighouse and Swift acknowledge, their appeal to the value of intimacy is inspired by Ferdinand Schoeman, "Rights of Children, Rights of Parents, and the Moral Basis of the Family," *Ethics* 91, no. 1 (October 1, 1980): 6–19.

[42] If so, then so much the worse for the Parental Influence objection. I don't pretend my brief responses to Feinberg- or Clayton-like views settle the matter. Clayton's development and defense of parental anti-perfectionism is detailed and subtle.

interests of their children. But it directs our attention to another painfully obvious point: parental influence doesn't play a huge role in shaping *all* of a child's future significant interests. There are some interests that a child will likely develop in spite of (possibly partly because of!) permissible parental influence. Children often develop interests and values that are very different from their parents' (sometimes to the consternation of their parents). In other words, we should distinguish between parentally influenced interests and non-parentally influenced interests. The distinction is not a sharp one. The true account of how a child developed a particular interest will usually appeal to (intentional) parental influence among many other, non-parental influences. Even so, there are interests a person is likely to develop no matter what permissible parental influencing takes place.

An interest in genetic knowledge is plausibly one such interest. A donor-conceived person is likely to develop a significant interest in having genetic knowledge no matter what his parents permissibly do to try to make him largely uninterested. The "permissibly" here is very important. We can imagine a futuristic hellscape where parents are able to directly manipulate the brains of their children so as to inculcate certain interests and not others. Parents could then directly influence (well, cause) children not to develop an interest in genetic knowledge. Back in the real world, some parents of donor-conceived children can quite reliably ensure their child does not develop a significant interest in searching for their donor by, for example, not telling their child she is donor-conceived.[43] So to claim that donor-conceived people are largely immune from parental influence when it comes to having an interest in genetic knowledge is not to suggest that there is *nothing* parents could do to shape their kids on this front. The claim, rather, is that using these forms of shaping is impermissible. And then the further implicit claim (which I'm now making explicit) is that no permissible form of influence is likely to prevent the child from developing a significant interest in genetic knowledge.

This is an empirical conjecture. But I think it is highly plausible. Facts about how children are conceived (i.e. that sperm and egg are required), plus the fact that the plurality of kids have both genetic parents raising them, plus whatever cultural forces push in the direction of suggesting that having

---

[43] Although if what I said in the previous chapter is right, these kids still probably have an interest in genetic knowledge. The idea, recall, is that non-disclosure likely doesn't prevent a donor-conceived person from *developing* the interest. Rather, it makes them believe it is already met (when, in fact, it is being frustrated).

genetic knowledge matters—*all* conspire to make the question "Who is my (other) genetic parent?" almost unavoidably of interest *at least* to children who do not know their complete genetic parentage. It is not entirely unavoidable; some donor-conceived people genuinely do not seem interested in the question. But it is a very good bet that any given donor-conceived person will be interested no matter what their parents permissibly do to make them uninterested.

I do not intend this last claim to express a kind of universal anthropological-*cum*-normative truth about human beings. My claim is that given the current practice of donor conception in the developed world—a world that largely operates with a genetics-based understanding of family and kin relations—it is a very good bet that any given donor-conceived person will be interested in having genetic knowledge. I do not claim that societies have *always* arranged childrearing and family structures in a way that is likely to make questions about genetic relatedness salient. Nor do I claim that they *should* always arrange themselves in this way. Suppose society changes so that most people simply don't care very much at all about genetic relatedness.[44] It could very well be that donor-conceived people in that society do *not* usually develop an interest in genetic knowledge. The Significant Interest view would have no purchase in such a world. So the Significant Interest view is not timeless. But it is not *meant* to be timeless. It is, rather, an argument for our world.

5. A larger challenge to the view

The Significant Interest view depends on the idea that satisfaction of a person's *worthwhile* significant interests makes their life go better. But I have said nothing to defend the idea that an interest in genetic knowledge is worthwhile even in the minimal sense I intend. In fact, my response to the Parental Influence objection might suggest that it isn't.

Here's why: I've claimed that given the world we live in, donor-conceived people are very likely to have a significant interest in genetic knowledge. But I also admitted that there is nothing inevitable—descriptively or normatively—about family structures that emphasize genetic relatedness. And this raises the possibility that people's interest in genetic knowledge is

---

[44] Really, we need to imagine that it changes in a *morally acceptable* way, i.e. that people's lack of interest in genetic knowledge isn't the result of mind manipulation or joining a massive cult or some such.

not worthwhile, not because it is trivial but because it is morally problematic. The full story of why it might be morally problematic unfolds in chapter 5, but the rough idea is easily explained.

Some might think the interest is morally problematic in virtue of evincing and entrenching a kind of bionormative prejudice according to which genetic ties—and family forms based on genetic ties—are of great significance (when they're not).[45] Inmaculada De Melo-Martín expresses this line of thought very nicely:

> Emphasizing the importance of genetic relationships might . . . encourage problematic beliefs about the superiority of biological families. . . . If emphasizing the importance of genetic information has the effect of idealizing the biological family, then it may actually undermine the interests of donor-conceived individuals.[46]

The morally problematic nature of the interest in genetic knowledge, on this view, might be likened to the way in which certain gendered interests are morally problematic, like the interest, perhaps, that some women have to conform to a certain conception of sexual attractiveness or the interest, perhaps, that some men have to conform to a certain conception of masculinity. These gendered interests reflect, and result from, deeply problematic societal structures and attitudes about men and women. We are not apt to blame individuals for having these interests. Indeed, we might think it is not only understandable but rational that they have these interests given their options. Even so, we will acknowledge that it would be best if the structures and attitudes that give rise to the interests were different. Moreover, we will wish that these interests did not arise so readily as live possibilities, let alone desirable or rational ones. If we could choose whether people have the interest and satisfy

---

[45] A version of this idea can be found in Charlotte Witt, "Family Resemblances: Adoption, Personal Identity, and Genetic Essentialism," in *Adoption Matters: Philosophical and Feminist Essays,* ed. Sally Haslanger and Charlotte Witt (Ithaca, NY: Cornell University Press, 2005), 265–90; Charlotte Witt, "Family, Self and Society: A Critique of the Bionormative Conception of the Family," in *Family-Making: Contemporary Ethical Challenges,* ed. Carolyn MacLeod and Françoise Baylis (New York: Oxford University Press, 2014); Haslanger, "Family, Ancestry, and Self"; Leighton, "Addressing the Harms of Not Knowing One's Heredity"; John B. Appleby and Anja Karnein, "On the Moral Importance of Genetic Ties in Families," in *Relatedness in Assisted Reproduction: Families, Origins and Identities,* ed. T. Freeman, F. Ebtehaj, S. Graham, and M. Richards (Cambridge: Cambridge University Press, 2014), 79–96; Inmaculada De Melo-Martín, "The Ethics of Anonymous Gamete Donation: Is There a Right to Know One's Genetic Origins?," *Hastings Center Report* 44, no. 2 (2014): 28–35.

[46] Melo-Martín, "The Ethics of Anonymous Gamete Donation," 33.

it or don't have the interest in the first place, we would choose the latter. This is a mark of the interest being morally problematic in the relevant sense. And the objection to the Significant Interest view is that the interest in genetic knowledge is morally problematic in just this sense.

This objection—which I call the Bionormativity objection—joins the Sideshow objection as an outstanding challenge to the Significant Interest view. The Sideshow objection, you'll recall, maintains that insofar as the Significant Interest view concedes that an interest in genetic knowledge is worthwhile, then the argument for using an open donor should go through claims about *what makes the interest worthwhile*, and not through the (supposedly) derivative fact that donor-conceived people tend to have a subjective interest in having genetic knowledge.

The two objections pull in different directions. One claims the Significant Interest view oversells the value of genetic knowledge. The other claims the Significant Interest view undersells the value of genetic knowledge. What is needed in response to *both* challenges is an account of the value of genetic knowledge, one that prevents the Significant Interest view from falling prey to either objection. Providing such an account is the work of the next two chapters.

4

The Value of Genetic Knowledge

The lost sequence in life, they say, is the thing we always search out.
—Michael Ondaatje, *Warlight*, 2018

There is a picture of an object to be searched out, the right kind, the kind that is true to nature, a fixed target if only we can get there.
—Ian Hacking, *The Social Construction of What?*, 1999

The Significant Interest view claims that intended parents have a weighty reason to use an open donor since it is foreseeable that a donor-conceived person is likely to develop a significant worthwhile interest in acquiring genetic knowledge.[1]

The view seems vulnerable to one of two very different objections. First, it appears that the Significant Interest view is parasitic on the claim that genetic knowledge *really matters,* that it has value apart from a person's subjective interest in it. After all, the Significant Interest view claims that a person's interest in genetic knowledge is *worthwhile.* But then, the objection goes, the Significant Interest view is a kind of sideshow: if a person's interest in acquiring genetic knowledge is worthwhile, then the case for using an open donor should go directly through the claim that having genetic knowledge is valuable and not through what appears to be a mere symptom of its value, namely that many people are actually interested in genetic knowledge.

The Sideshow objection is motivated by the thought that the Significant Interest view undersells the value of genetic knowledge. The second objection is motivated by the thought that the Significant Interest view *oversells* its value. According to the second objection, the idea that an interest

---

[1] To say that parents have a weighty reason to use an open donor doesn't show that they have a *decisive* reason. Perhaps other considerations, when added to the mix, show that intended parents don't have reason to use an identity release donor all things considered. I return to this issue in chapter 6.

Conceiving People. Daniel Groll, Oxford University Press. © Oxford University Press 2021.
DOI: 10.1093/oso/9780190063054.003.0004

in acquiring genetic knowledge is worthwhile *at all* is suspect. People's interest in acquiring genetic knowledge could be trivial[2] or, worse, morally problematic in virtue of evincing a kind of bionormative prejudice, i.e. a set of attitudes and practices that unjustifiably valorize genetic ties and the bionormative family. I say a lot more about what that means—and whether it is true—in the next chapter. The idea now is that *if* it is true, then the idea that parents have any obligation to help their children satisfy an interest in genetic knowledge is highly suspect.

Considered in tandem, the objections suggest that the Significant Interest view is unstable. It either collapses into the view that having genetic knowledge really matters or it dissolves altogether. This chapter and the next deal with these objections. In this chapter, I take on the Sideshow objection. I offer an account of the value of genetic knowledge according to which it is a *prudentially optional good*. It is a prudential good because it can (and often does) play a crucial role in an activity with profound prudential value: healthy identity determination. But it is *optional* because healthy identity determination does not require that one pursue the "genetic route," as I call it; other routes are available and they are not second best to the genetic route.[3]

The argument for this view has two corollaries. First, the Profound Prudential Good view—according to which genetic knowledge has non-optional, universal, weighty importance—is mistaken. Second, the Significant Interest view is not a sideshow. An appeal to the actual interests of donor-conceived people is crucial for showing that intended parents should use an open donor.

---

[2] Bearing in mind that we are setting aside the Medical Reasons view.

[3] Versions of this idea are in Charlotte Witt, "Family Resemblances: Adoption, Personal Identity, and Genetic Essentialism," in *Adoption Matters: Philosophical and Feminist Essays*, ed. Charlotte Witt and Sally Haslanger (Ithaca, NY: Cornell University Press, 2005), 265–90; Sally Haslanger, "Family, Ancestry, and Self," in *Resisting Reality: Social Construction and Social Critique* (New York: Oxford University Press, 2012), 158–182; Hallvard Lillehammer, "Who Cares Where You Come from? Cultivating Virtues of Indifference," in *Relatedness in Assisted Reproduction: Families, Origins and Identities*, ed. T. Freeman et al. (Cambridge: Cambridge University Press, 2014), 97–112. I deploy and acknowledge that work in what follows. My account of the value of genetic knowledge is by no means complete. With the exception of a small paragraph below, I say almost nothing about people's interest in ancestry. And I say nothing about the interest many parents—including the parents of donor-conceived children—have in raising a child that is at least partly genetically related to them. However, I think much of what I say below could be redeployed to explain this interest (at least in part).

1. Chauvinism versus pluralism

I like music a lot. It would be a personal calamity if someone told me I couldn't listen to or play music again. But lots of people aren't really into music. It's not that they don't like it. It's just that they don't really pay any attention to it. Listening, let alone playing, music isn't an important part of their lives. Their relationship to music is like mine to painting. It's not that I don't like engaging with paintings. But I spend more or less no time doing so (and actually trying to paint doesn't interest me in the least). I wouldn't be too bothered if someone told me I could never behold another painting.[4]

What to make of this? Am I missing something genuinely valuable by not being interested in painting? Are you missing something genuinely valuable by not being interested in music? I am inclined to answer "yes" to both questions. But there are two strengths, to to speak, that the "yes" answer might take:

1. **The chauvinistic "yes"**: Your life is *impoverished* by your lack of interest in music and mine is *impoverished* by my lack of interest in painting. To say one's life is "impoverished" is to say that it is worse in a way that cannot be compensated for by the presence of other goods. For example, not being interested in music is akin to not being interested in friendship, and a life without friends is significantly impoverished. A life without friendship lacks a profound prudential good, and other goods cannot compensate for its lack.[5]

---

[4] Setting aside the issue of what such a situation would imply about the state of the world or my place in it.

[5] This formulation of the view—and the Profound Prudential Good view in general—is meant to capture Velleman's thought that while lacking genetic knowledge is a serious impoverishment in one's life, it does *not* preclude those that lack it from having lives worth living or even flourishing lives. But now one might wonder: If that's the case—if lives that lack genetic knowledge can be (well) worth living—what objection could there be to creating such lives? Velleman's answer is that the threshold for permissibly *creating* a life is considerably higher than that life (merely) being worth living. In other words, a life that lacks X might be (well) worth living, but intentionally *creating* a life that will lack X is impermissible. This is because it evinces a lack of respect for the kind of thing you are creating, i.e. a person. It is disrespectful, on this view, because the alternative to creating the "truncated" life, namely non-existence, is in no way a *harm* to the potential person. Given that it is not a harm, the bar for creating the life is high. If you're going to bring someone into existence, you best ensure that their life will not lack for highly important goods (even if lives without those goods are worth living). If you think having genetic knowledge is a highly important good, intentionally creating someone who will lack it does not clear the bar for permissible procreation. But once someone exists, it may be best for the person—and fully compatible with respecting them—to put them up for adoption, for example, since doing so is overall a benefit to them. So Velleman is not committed to the view that putting a child up for adoption (without giving them access to genetic knowledge) is impermissible on the grounds that the child will be deprived of a profound prudential good. Even so, he is clearly committed to the idea that lacking genetic knowledge puts one at a significant disadvantage with

2. The pluralistic "yes": There is something genuinely valuable about music and something genuinely valuable about painting. As a result, it is true that the person who is not interested in painting is really missing something; there is some domain of genuine value to which they are insensitive. But their life is not thereby *impoverished*. For example, a lack of engagement with painting can be compensated for by an engagement with music.

The pluralistic view doesn't maintain that music and painting are fungible. If it did, then it would be strange to think that the person who is interested in painting, but not music, is missing something (in the same way it would be strange to think that someone who has a $100 bill is missing something in virtue of having *this* $100 bill rather than *that* $100 bill). The pluralistic view maintains that you *are* missing something because the good of music is not the same as the good of painting and vice versa.

But then why can one compensate for the other? One answer is that they are instances, or specifications, of some more general good, something like the good of *creative activity*. A life that lacks creative activity altogether is lacking something profoundly prudentially good. People should have creative activity in their lives. But whether that activity takes the form of engaging with music or painting or crocheting or dB drag-racing is, other things being equal, not of great importance (at least prudentially speaking). Of course, it might be of tremendous importance for a particular person that she engages with music and not dB drag-racing. But this is not because engaging with music, as such, is a non-optional prudential good. Engaging in creative activity is the non-optional prudential good. After that, people have options. That doesn't mean that the creative activity a person pursues is a matter of radical choice. Some combination of taste, opportunity, personality, talent and luck will push people down one path rather than another. But from the point of view of engaging with something that matters, there are choices.[6]

---

respect to doing well at a crucial component of flourishing, namely determining one's identity. That is the point I take issue with in this chapter. J. David Velleman, "III. Love and Nonexistence," *Philosophy & Public Affairs* 36, no. 3 (2008): 266–88.

[6] Dan Moller, "Wealth, Disability, and Happiness," *Philosophy & Public Affairs* (2011): vol. 2, 198–99.

My goal is not to adjudicate between the chauvinistic view and pluralistic view when it comes to music and painting. The point I am making is this: it is possible to think that something is genuinely valuable without thinking that a life without it is thereby impoverished.

My account of the value of genetic knowledge turns on this possibility. I maintain that having genetic knowledge is genuinely valuable. Its value is not fungible, but a life that lacks it is not thereby impoverished.[7] Genetic knowledge is an optional prudential good. Moreover, it is possible to value it as such. Someone who *loves* music, who cannot imagine her life without it, and who thinks that it is objectively valuable, can acknowledge that the lives of people who have no real interest in music are not thereby impoverished. So too someone who thinks that genetic knowledge is objectively valuable, who has built her life around it, and cannot imagine her life without it, can acknowledge that the lives of people who lack genetic knowledge (and who have no real interest in having it) are not thereby impoverished.

In other words: thinking that genetic knowledge is valuable need not commit one to *genetic chauvinism*. Someone who has structured her life around music need not think that the musical life is more valuable than the painterly life, that it provides *the* model for what an artistic life looks like. Likewise, someone who has structured his life in a way that depends on valuing genetic relatedness needn't see families that are structured around such relatedness as having more value than other kinds of family structures, as providing *the* model for what a family should be.

At this point, I want to remind you of something from chapter 1: when I talk about "genetic knowledge" I mean knowledge of who one's genetic progenitors are and not, more broadly, ancestral genetic knowledge (e.g. knowledge of who your [genetic] grandparents or great-grandparents are). Many people value ancestral genetic knowledge. But the account I give of the value of genetic knowledge focuses more narrowly on knowing who your genetic parents are.

You might think an account that explains the value of (progenitor) genetic knowledge can be extended to show that ancestral genetic knowledge is valuable as well. Maybe. Some of what I say about the value of genetic knowledge—in particular, the story I tell about the importance to some people of answering the question "How did I come to be?" with genetic

---

[7] The Profound Prudential Good view is chauvinistic. It maintains that a life that lacks genetic knowledge is thereby impoverished.

knowledge—could be used to offer a limited account of the value of ancestral knowledge. But I am considerably less confident that other parts of the story I tell can be used in the same way.

Whether or not it can is not my concern. Instead, my overall argument depends on the more modest (and, in my view, more defensible) claim that knowing who your genetic parents are is prudentially valuable. And so, in what follows, keep in mind that "genetic knowledge" means "knowledge of who your genetic parents are."

But why think that genetic knowledge even in that more limited sense is valuable? To sharpen the question, consider music and painting once more. A life that is not engaged with music but is engaged with painting is not thereby impoverished because both music and painting are instantiations of some more general good: artistic activity. There are substantial questions about what the relevant, more general category is, how to delineate it, and whether it has pluralistic or chauvinistic objective value. But I don't think anything turns on how we answer these questions. Indeed, some might reject the idea that music and painting are plural goods, thinking instead that they are chauvinistic goods. That's fine too. This person can simply choose more fine-grained categories. Even if music is a chauvinistic good, surely particular genres of music (hip hop versus country) are not.

The point I am after is this: *wherever* one locates a pluralistic good, there will be some more general good to which the pluralistic good belongs as one instantiation among others of the more general good. So to make the case that genetic knowledge is a plural good, we need to know which more general good it is a specification of. If "genetic knowledge" is analogous to "music," what plays the role of "artistic activity" in the analogy?

We have already seen the answer in the brief discussion of the Profound Prudential Good view in chapter 3. The fundamental claim of the Profound Prudential Good view is that genetic knowledge is necessary, or nearly so, for healthy identity determination.[8] I argue below that we should reject this strong claim. But we should accept the weaker claim that genetic knowledge is valuable for the role it can play in healthy identity determination.[9]

---

[8] I have chosen this word deliberately since "determination" is ambiguous between an epistemic activity and what I call an "agential" activity. I say a lot about this below (pp. 112–16).

[9] Beyond whatever medical value it has. As we'll see, my understanding of what falls under the umbrella of "identity determination" is quite broad and encompasses ways of forging and understanding connections to genetic progenitors. Thanks to Rivka Weinberg for pushing me on this point.

2. Healthy identity determination: answering the question "Who am I?"

Katrina Clark is a donor-conceived person. When she was 17, she found out who her genetic father is. She explains her feelings upon seeing a picture of him for the first time:

> From my computer screen, my own face seemed to stare back at me. And just like that, after 17 years, the missing piece of the puzzle snapped into place. The puzzle of who I am.[10]

The question "Who am I?" is one that occurs again and again in accounts of why donor-conceived people search for their genetic parents. The person who asks it is engaged in the task of identity determination.

But what exactly is that task? What are we wondering when we ask "Who am I?" Katrina Clark, no doubt, already knew a *lot* about who she is. She is not like the Hollywood amnesiac who has literally forgotten key facts about herself (her name, whether she is married, her occupation, who her friends are, *etc.*). So, what is someone like Katrina, or indeed any of us non-amnesiacs, asking when we wonder "Who am I?"

I maintain that the question "Who am I?" can be deconstructed into the following three questions, which I call *the identity questions*:

1. What am I (like)? (What are my features or traits?)
2. Who am I like? (Whom do I resemble?)
3. How am I? (How did *I* come to be? How did history go so as to produce *me*, i.e. this particular individual?)

Thinking of identity determination in terms of answering the identity questions—or indeed, even just in terms of the question "Who am I?"—threatens to over-intellectualize the task. Most people probably do not sharply differentiate between, let alone explicitly ask themselves, these questions (although certainly some do). Rather, we provide ourselves

---

[10] Katrina Clark, "Who's Your Daddy?," *Washington Post*, December 17, 2006, https://www.washingtonpost.com/archive/opinions/2006/12/17/whos-your-daddy/856d8f09-d17c-4a0c-be1b-5435190b084c/. I came across this particular quotation in Naomi R. Cahn, *The New Kinship: Constructing Donor-Conceived Families* (New York: NYU Press, 2013), 76.

with answers whenever we look in a mirror, or think "I'm not very good at dancing," or say "I am *so* like my mother."

In thinking of ourselves in some terms rather than others, we are developing a picture of who we are or what Oyersman et al. call a *self-concept*: "what comes to mind when one thinks of oneself, one theory of one's personality, and what one believes is true of oneself."[11] The goal is not just to develop *any* sense of self, but rather one that reflects how you actually are, what is *true* of oneself. In other words, identity determination is not just a phenomenological task, a matter of developing a coherent self-concept whatever it may be. Someone who is convinced he is Napoleon might have a coherent self-concept and, indeed, maybe have a very robust sense of identity phenomenologically speaking. But in a straightforward way, he does not know who he is. Less dramatically, the blowhard who believes he is a good listener or the selfish friend who thinks she is especially giving might have coherent self-concepts, but they, too, do not know who they are. Identity determination is geared toward genuine self-understanding, toward an answer to the question "Who am I?" that is grounded in how things are.

The identity questions are not all concerned with the same sense of "identity." Talk of "identity" often conflates two distinct senses of the term.[12] Sometimes when we (at least philosophers) talk about identity, we have in mind features of a person that make her the *kind* of person she is. You say: "Tell me about Chickie. I want to know who he is." I say: "Chickie is a professor and a father. He is tall and balding. He is opinionated, ornery, and obnoxious. He loves whisky. That's Chickie!" I've told you a little about what Chickie is like. I have given you a sense of what I will call his *kind identity*, i.e. what features make him the kind of individual he is.[13]

A person's kind identity can change. Suppose Chickie suffers an unfortunate tongue injury that causes him to hate the taste of whisky. He is so depressed by this turn of events that he stops turning up to work and is fired.

---

[11] Daphna Oyserman et al., "Self, Self-Concept and Identity," in *Handbook of Self and Identity*, ed. Mark R. Leary and June Price Tangney (New York: Guilford Press, 2012), 69. Citations removed from the quotation.

[12] Both Witt, "Family Resemblances" and Lillehammer, "Who Cares Where You Come From?" discuss these senses of identity in connection to genetic relatedness.

[13] Witt calls this "personal identity." Witt, "Family Resemblances," 140. Lillehammer calls it "practical identity." Lillehammer, "Who Cares Where You Come From?," 100. The discussion here might make it sound as though each person has one, specific identity to discover. But that's not right for reasons I explain in a little bit. The features of a person constrain what counts as an acceptable answer to the question "What is this person's individual identity?," but they do not by themselves determine the person's identity.

A hollow shell of his former self, Chickie stops socializing and keeps his opinions to himself. When you say to me now "Tell me about Chickie," my answer will be different. But I'll still be talking about *Chickie*; the one and the same person has undergone a change. Now-Chickie is metaphysically identical to Then-Chickie. His *kind* identity has undergone a serious change, but his metaphysical identity has not. He has not literally ceased to exist.

The first two questions—"What am I (like)?" and "Who am I like?"—are concerned with *kind* identity. The person who asks them is interested in what features she has and who else has those features. The third question—"How am I?"—is concerned with metaphysical identity. The person who asks this question is interested in how events conspired to produce *him* metaphysically speaking: "How is it," he asks, "that *I* came to be born? What series of events made me exist rather than someone else?" The focus here is not on how he came to be the kind of person he is but on how he came to be *at all* (no matter what kind of person he is).

The upshot is that someone who asks "Who am I?" could be concerned with two different tasks. She might be interested in determining something about her kind identity or she might be interested in determining something about her metaphysical identity. What this means is that general claims about the place of genetic knowledge in healthy identity determination need to be scrutinized. In particular, we need to know: What is the place of genetic knowledge in determining one's identity in either sense?

3. "How am I?"

Let's start with the question "How am I?" since it seems the most amenable to having genetic knowledge play a privileged role in the answer. A person's interest in how their genetic parents met plausibly reflects an interest in this question: "How did you two come to be together such that I resulted (for had you not come together, *I* would not have resulted)?" More generally, a person's interest in their ancestry at least sometimes reflects an interest in the question "How am I?" For example, I might say to myself, "Had my grandparents not left Lithuania, my father never would have met my mother and I would not have been born!" The interest here is not in what kind of person I am, but in the fact that *I am* at all. Knowing your genetic parentage is knowing a metaphysically necessary condition for your existence. You could not have been born to other parents. Perhaps someone like you would exist, but not you. Another way of putting this is that, unlike the fact that your hair is cut short or that you are six feet tall, the fact that your genetic parents are Gail and Melvin is not a contingent feature of you. No other people could have been your genetic parents.

Now this answer to the "How am I?" question is something you (can) know without knowing who your genetic parents are. In other words: a general answer to the question, "How did I come to be?" doesn't require having genetic knowledge of the sort we are interested in.

But at least some versions of a more specific answer do. It is easy to imagine someone who wants to have a narrative, a fairly detailed picture, of how the world went so as to produce them. And as part of that more specific narrative, they may want to know, "Whose gametes got together? And how? And why?"

The "How" question can be answered for a donor-conceived person without genetic knowledge. It is enough to know how donor conception works. It is also possible to have an answer to the "Why" question without knowing who the donor is. Perhaps the donor bequeathed the donor-conceived child's parents a letter explaining his rationale for donating. But if an anonymous donor does not do this, or something like it, then a largely complete answer to the "Why?" question is foreclosed to the resulting person.

Without a doubt, though, the first question, "*Whose* gametes got together?," cannot be answered without genetic knowledge, at least not on the most natural interpretation of the question. The person who asks "Whose gametes am I the product of?" wants more of an answer than "My mother Estrella and Donor 768452." They want to know who Donor 768452 *is*. Perhaps they would like to know what he looks like (but not as a way of answering the "What am I [like]?" or "Who am I like?" questions—we'll get to those questions in due time). Rather, they want a somewhat fleshed-out picture of the progression of events and actors that led to their coming to be. A donor number will not be enough; they want a face and a name. They want genetic knowledge.

The point here is not just to register the fact that some people want to know the identity of their genetic parents. Rather, it is that one way to see this interest as worthwhile is because it provides an answer to the question "How am I?" A real-life version of a partly genetics-based answer to the question "How am I?" comes from Kevin Walters, who, in 2014, chained himself to the Des Plaines Oasis—a highway rest stop outside of Chicago—to protest its destruction. Here's why:

"About 21 years ago, my parents were at a Phil Collins concert here in Chicago, and one thing led to another. They ended up at the oasis . . . and I was conceived there," he said. . . . Walters said the oasis is part of his life, and he hates to see it close.[14]

Walters, clearly, is interested in the details of his conception, which includes not only knowledge of his genetic and social parents, but also some of the details of exactly when and how he was conceived. His answer to the question "How am I?" turns on having genetic knowledge (as well as some Phil Collins–based knowledge). Now, it's hard not to see Walters' protest as at least partly tongue-in-cheek. Nonetheless it reflects, however histrionically, an interest that a lot of people have in knowing how circumstances conspired to give rise to *them*.

But having genetic knowledge is certainly not necessary for knowing that. After all, all kinds of events had to transpire in just the way they did for it to have been the case that you were born. If your mother had missed her bus, she wouldn't have met your father. If your grandparents had not left Lithuania in 1921, they would have been killed with the rest of their family in the Holocaust (and so your father would not have been born and so you would not have been born). There are so many ways in which things had to unfold just as they did so as to produce you. The upshot is that no one has a complete answer to the question "How am I?" The problem is not just that most of the facts that would figure into a complete answer are lost to history. The problem is also that all narratives must leave stuff out. In determining an answer to the question "How am I?," choices must be made. The story will focus on certain preconditions of our existence and leave out others altogether (even if one knows about them). Some will be treated as crucial to the narrative, others as not worth mentioning at all.

The key claim is this: a perfectly good answer to the question need not treat the identity of the donor as relevant. A donor-conceived child's answer might emphasize the history of how her mothers met: "If Louise had decided not to accompany her friend Lester that night in Chicago to Schubas to see his friend Edith's set, Louise would not have met Edith, they would not have married, they would not have decided to have a child . . . and then no me!

---

[14] CBS Chicago, "Man Conceived at Des Plaines Oasis Stages One-Man Protest of Closure," March 14, 2014, https://chicago.cbslocal.com/2014/03/14/man-conceived-at-des-plaines-oasis-stages-one-man-protest-of-closure/.

That is how I came to be." When this donor-conceived person (accurately) pictures the unfolding of events that led to her, the identity of the donor is not remotely central.

The way in which an answer to the question "How am I?" can centrally turn on non-genetic facts is beautifully illustrated in a story by Emily Yoffe about her young daughter discovering that her father (Yoffe's husband) had a first wife who died several years into the marriage. Yoffe's daughter learns this at age 8 when she discovers a box of photos from her father's first marriage in the attic of her house:

> She brought [the photos] downstairs to our bedroom and said she wanted to look at the old pictures of Daddy. She asked about the pretty, dark-haired woman always standing next to him. My husband told her that was Robin. After a few more minutes she looked up and said, "There are so many pictures of her."
>
> "Dad loved her," I said.
>
> "If you loved her so much, why didn't you marry her?" she asked her father.
>
> He looked at me, and I nodded.
>
> "I did," he replied.
>
> Our daughter looked at the picture she was holding in her hand, her eyes widening, then at me. It was like one of those moments in Dickens when a foundling discovers her true origins.
>
> "It's like I have two mothers," she said in a kind of astonishment.
>
> I liked her formulation. And I thought Robin would be satisfied with how well her wish for her husband, now mine, had been fulfilled.
>
> My husband and I have been married for 15 years, more than twice as long as he was married to Robin. My daughter is 13 now and long ago outgrew the chair that Robin's family gave her. I keep it stored safely with her bassinet, the clown rattle, and her favorite jacket printed with elephants. I hope someday a granddaughter might use these things. If so, when that little girl is old enough, I will tell her the story of her other grandmother, Robin.[15]

---

[15] Emily Yoffe, "My Husband's Other Wife: She Died, So I Could Find the Man I Love," *Slate*, June 16, 2009, https://slate.com/human-interest/2009/06/my-husbands-other-wife-she-died-so-i-could-find-the-man-i-love.html.

This story is remarkable in a number of ways. It shows that even young children can be interested in the question "How am I?" Yoffe's daughter immediately keys into the fact that she would not exist had Robin not died. Moreover, Yoffe's daughter's reaction—"It's like I have two mothers!"—shows that non-genetic preconditions of one's existence can play a significant part in someone's story of how they came to be. Indeed, facts about genetic relatedness may play no significant role at all for someone in answering the question "How am I?" They may be left on the cutting-room floor of the person's narrative. The upshot is that accurately answering the question "How am I?" *via* the genetic route is optional: it is one way of engaging in (part of) the task of healthy identity determination. Acquiring the knowledge is prudentially valuable, but nonetheless optional.

One might respond to this line of thought by pointing out that it fails to acknowledge a difference between, on the one hand, such facts as "Had my father's first wife lived, I would not exist" and, on the other hand, "Had my parents' genetic material never combined, I would not exist." The second claim is modally stronger. It is not metaphysically possible for you to exist had your genetic parents' gametes never combined. But it is possible that you would have existed even if your father's first wife had lived. He might have met your genetic mother anyway and they might have conceived you at exactly the same time and the very same sperm might have met the very same egg. It is vanishingly unlikely. But it is possible.

What should we make of this? Does the fact that genetic answers to the question "How am I?" involve a kind of necessity that at least some non-genetic answers lack make the genetic answer more significant, more of a "real" answer, than the non-genetic one?

No doubt some people will be moved by the fact that metaphysical necessity attaches to facts about who your genetic parents are, but not to facts about making it to the bus on time. They will see it as significant that, metaphysically speaking, there is at least one point in history leading to them that *could not have gone differently*. As a result, building an answer to the question "How am I?" largely around that point might well be very important to them.

But others might not be moved by this line of thought at all. They might acknowledge that there is a difference in the kind of necessity that attaches to the genetic story and the non-genetic story. But they may simply not treat that difference as significant. "Of course," a donor-conceived person might say, "I would not be me had my mother's egg not combined with Donor

546792's sperm. Some version of that is true of *everyone*. What I find fascinating, when I think about how I came to be, is the fortuitousness of how my mothers met."

So who is right? The question is not a fruitful one. Both paths are acceptable. Whether one privileges a genetic answer to the question "How am I?" is a choice point in the task of identity determination. That is, independent of a person's interest one way or the other, it is indeterminate whether a genetic answer to the question "How am I?" is more significant than a non-genetic answer. It is, roughly, a matter of taste, not unlike a preference for music over painting. Some people will be deeply moved by the genetic answer. For them, knowing the identity of their genetic parents might matter deeply as part of answering the question "How am I?" Moreover, they are not mistaken in caring about it so much, just as the person who is deeply invested in music is not mistaken in caring about it so much. But someone who thinks the difference in metaphysical strength between the genetic and non-genetic answers is utterly irrelevant, and so emphasizes the latter instead of the former in answering the question "How am I?," is not making a mistake. You only make a mistake if you have a *chauvinistic* attitude about the significance or insignificance of the genetic answer to the question "How am I?"

4. "What am I (like)?"

Once past infancy, and barring serious cognitive disabilities, we all have some self-conception, some set of answers to the question "What am I (like)?" This self-conception will include beliefs about many different aspects of ourselves. Some will be about the roles we occupy: I am a father. I am a philosophy professor. Others will be about our physical attributes: I am slender. I have a big nose. Still others will be about our personality: I am impatient. I am organized. I love music.

We already know that genuine identity determination must be at least minimally responsive to the facts.[16] One way it can fail in this regard is by being constituted in significant ways by false beliefs or delusions.[17] Think again of our Napoleon. Or consider a less pathological example:

---

[16] See (p. 88).
[17] Richard Dub, "Delusions, Acceptances, and Cognitive Feelings," *Philosophy and Phenomenological Research* 94, no. 1 (2017): 27–60.

88Self-absorbed Richard: Richard thinks he is good at comforting friends in need. He thinks does an excellent job listening to people and giving them what they need in the moment, whether it be sympathy or suggestions or just a shoulder to cry on. It is one of the things he is most proud of about himself. In reality, Richard always makes discussions about other people's challenges and problems about him. Everyone (except Richard) knows that no matter where the conversation begins, it will end with Richard talking about himself.[18]

Inasmuch as Richard is settled in a false belief about what he is like, he is failing to genuinely determine his identity.

But one can fail at the task of identity determination by simply *lacking* important information about oneself—think again of the Hollywood amnesiac. To the extent that he cannot recover very basic facts about himself, he will struggle, mightily, at determining his identity. More generally, simply being unable to acquire significant information about what we are like can get in the way of healthy identity determination.

How should we think of information about one's genetic parentage in this context? It is often assumed that genetic knowledge plays a central role, that it is a source of substantial self-knowledge with respect to the question of what one *is* like or what one *will be* like (or more weakly, what one is *inclined* to be like). Having genetic knowledge is often compared to looking in a mirror:

> One's genetic heritage is evident in one's appearance, temperament, interests, abilities and other traits. In this sense, biologically based experiences of the self are core parts of one's identity.
>
> People deprived of knowledge of their progenitors . . . have lost this important component of self-knowledge. [. . .] The absence of a mirror [in the form of one's genetic progenitors] and the opportunity to see oneself in one's biological ties hinders identity formation for the donor-conceived.[19]

---

[18] All of us are prone to self-deception to some extent. We think we are better drivers than we are; smarter than we are; less prone to various cognitive biases than we are. We are, then, to some extent, failing at the task of identity determination (even if being self-deceived to some extent is, overall, good for us).

[19] J. Benward et al., "Identity Development in the Donor-Conceived Child," in *The Right to Know One's Origins: Assisted Human Reproduction and the Best Interests of Children,* ed. Juliet Ruth Guichon, Ian Mitchell, and Michelle Giroux (Brussels: ASP, 2012), 167.

Just as I can learn a lot about how I look from looking in a mirror, so too I can learn a lot about myself from knowing my genetic origins. The idea is that someone who is cut off from knowledge of their genetic origins is cut off from an important source of self-knowledge, knowledge of what they are like.

The interest in accessing this purported source of self-knowledge goes beyond learning simple, or bare, facts about your appearance (after all, you could just look in the mirror). Rather, the idea is that one can access subtler, harder-to-discern facts about yourself from seeing another who is genetically close to you. As Velleman puts it:

> If I want to see myself as another . . . I don't have to imagine myself as seen through the other people's eyes: I just have to look at my father, my mother, and my brothers, who show me by way of family resemblance, what I am like. For information about my appearance, they may not be as good a source as an ordinary mirror; but for information about what I am like as a person, they are the closest thing to a mirror that I can find.[20]

According to Velleman, knowing what kind of person we are, what our kind identity is, amounts to having a literal "family-resemblance concept,"[21] the

> concept for the personal type of which I happen to be the only instance but to which a *Doppelgänger* would belong, if I had one. I would recognize a *Doppelganger* under this concept, by our family resemblance.[22]

The crucial point for Velleman is that:

> Forming a useful family-resemblance concept of myself would be very difficult were I not acquainted with people to whom I bear a literal family resemblance. Knowing what I am like would be that much harder if I didn't know other people like me.[23]

Velleman writes in the first person, but he clearly thinks that what is true for him is true for more or less everybody: we all will have a hard time answering

[20] J. David Velleman, "Family History," *Philosophical Papers* 34, no. 3 (2005): 368.
[21] Velleman, "Family History," 365.
[22] Velleman, "Family History," 365.
[23] Velleman, "Family History," 366.

the question "What am I like?" without being acquainted with our genetic families.

It is worth looking closely at the mirror metaphor. Even if Velleman is right that we need a mirror in the form of other people to know what we are like, it is not clear why we need a *genetic* mirror (so to speak) to know what we are like. As Haslanger puts it:

> We all rely on many sources in our development of self-understanding, including friends, characters in literature and film, public figures and, in cases where biological kin are missing, custodial family members. If the crucial thing is that we have others around us who effectively mirror us to ourselves, then it isn't clear why this should be a biological relative.[24]

The obvious response to this line of thought is that our genetic relatives are most likely to be most like us. So if we are looking for a mirror in the form of other people, we should look first to our genetic family for the most accurate mirror.

But this response—as intuitive as it might seem—allows us to see why the metaphor of the mirror threatens to mislead in more fundamental ways. One thing about a mirror is that you don't antecedently need to have any real idea of what you look like in order to know that the reflection you see is yours. You just need to know that a mirror faithfully reflects your image back at you. If the mirror shows someone with brown hair when you step in front of it, you can usually safely infer that you have brown hair.[25] You can go from knowing more or less nothing about the particulars of what you look like to having a pretty complete picture of what you look like by stepping in front of a mirror, so long as you roughly understand the mechanism at work.

Consider now the "mirror" of genetic knowledge. In order to make things clearer, let's suppose that the kind of genetic knowledge a donor-conceived person is interested in acquiring is knowledge by acquaintance. The donor-conceived person wants to see their genetic parent up close and interact with them so that they can know the person with a fineness of grain that merely reading a description won't provide. They want to see that the genetic parent

---

[24] Haslanger, "Family, Ancestry, and Self," 169.
[25] Some features of mirrors will lead you astray if you don't know how they work (or even if you do!).

has certain physical features, certain behavioral features, and certain personality features *in just these particular ways.*

To what extent is accessing this genetic knowledge akin to looking in a mirror? It depends on which features of the genetic parent we are focused on. Certain physical features—like the color of the person's eyes—can allow some generally safe inferences about the color of one's own eyes. More generally, the mirror metaphor works best when we focus on features of a person that are largely insensitive to non-genetic factors:[26] whether your earlobes are attached, whether you can do that thing with your tongue, the color of your eyes, whether you have freckles.[27] In other words, if someone has some basic knowledge of how genetic transmission works to replicate features of the genetic parents in the child, then the child can learn a lot about herself with respect to these features by being acquainted with her genetic parents. She doesn't need to have antecedent knowledge of how she looks (with respect to these features) in order to know that what she sees in her genetic parents is likely reflected back in her.

But as we move away entirely, or largely, from simple physical traits to more complex, subtle behavioral and personality traits, the mirror metaphor increasingly distorts. This is because the inferences someone can make about what they are like with respect to these traits *just* on the basis of knowing "These people are my genetic parents" become increasingly uncertain because the kind of direct genetic story that usually does the trick for eye color or that tongue thing, for example, doesn't apply for more complex behavioral and personality traits. It is true that our genetics set the boundaries for what traits we can have. But once we move past simple physical traits, the options available within the boundaries are large indeed. Consider physical traits like height, or weight, or gait. Clearly, genetics play a role in determining these things, but the interaction between genes and the environment allows for wide phenotypical variability.[28] The same is true with respect to behavioral features like laughing a certain way or speaking with a certain cadence.

---

[26] I am indebted to Ned Hall for a very helpful exchange on how to think, and best talk about, the causal contribution of genetics to phenotypical traits.

[27] Although even these examples are not really that straightforward. See http://learn.genetics.utah.edu/content/basics/observable/.

[28] Moreover, attempts to precisely apportion how much of genes versus environment (leaving aside that the very units of comparison are not well-defined) are responsible for a person's phenotypical traits is a conceptually confused task. See Evelyn Fox Keller, *The Mirage of a Space between Nature and Nurture* (Durham, NC: Duke University Press, 2010); Ned Hall, "Causal Contribution," in *Measuring the Global Burden of Disease: Philosophical Dimensions*, ed. Nir Eyal et al. (New York: Oxford University Press, 2020), 204–226.

And it is *clearly* true with respect to personality traits. Once we move beyond phenotypic traits that are largely insensitive to environmental influence, acquaintance with a genetic parent (even both genetic parents) does not by itself warrant inferences that are certain enough to provide anything like self-knowledge.[29]

This doesn't mean that there is nothing to learn. As Velleman emphasizes, seeing another who is like you with respect to some features can allow you to get a perspective on those features which is otherwise hard to get. It is hard for us to watch ourselves navigating the world from a third-person perspective. There are times when we are able to see ourselves from above, so to speak, to observe or reflect on what we are like. But the activity of doing this—of projecting ourselves into a third-person point of view of ourselves—tends to be self-conscious which, in turn, affects the very activity we are trying to observe.[30] We turn to face ourselves, but never catch a glimpse.[31] Interacting with someone who is like you can give you an opportunity to catch a glimpse of yourself you would not otherwise get. And inasmuch as your genetic progenitor is like you in some respects, then knowing your genetic progenitor can be a source of self-knowledge about what you are like.

But notice that this only works to the extent that you already have a pretty good idea of what you are like.[32] If you did not already know that this person is in your mold (or you are in their mold) then the fact that they do things this way, or move in that way, or deal with problems in this way won't teach you anything about yourself *even if* the person's behavior accurately reflects a part of you back at yourself. Velleman gets the connection between the formation of his family-resemblance concept and self-knowledge backward. Once we move beyond simple forms of resemblance, the formation of the family-resemblance concept (at least a rationally formed one) presupposes that the members have enough of a grasp of themselves to be able to see the other and say, "Hey! You resemble me in these ways!"

---

[29] I think there is a tendency—and I would say that it is on display in Velleman's piece—to oversimplify the genetic story so that people are inclined to explain a complex personality trait, e.g. fretting in the face of simple challenges, in terms of a simple genetic story ("My [genetic] mother is like that too! Genetics!"). This is a form of genetic essentialism according to which what I am like is almost entirely a function of, or at least is very tightly constrained by, my genetics.

[30] Velleman, "Family History," 366–67.

[31] With apologies to David Bowie.

[32] As Haslanger puts it: "[I]f you don't have some self-knowledge prior to seeing others like yourself, then how could you tell whether they are like you or not? After all: you don't know what you are like!" Haslanger, "Family, Ancestry, and Self," 169–70.

So, the role for genetic knowledge in answering the question "What am I like?" is more limited than it initially appeared. The features of me that I really can learn something about just on the basis of acquiring genetic knowledge are rather limited. Moreover, they are precisely those features that are easiest to learn about in other ways. The features I am in the best position to learn something new about simply by acquiring genetic knowledge are simple physical features. Ironically these can be effectively learned about by looking in a literal mirror (or looking at a photograph or watching a video). Contrariwise, the features that are more plausible candidates for being central to my conception of what I am like are ones that I am not well-positioned to learn something substantial about simply by gaining genetic knowledge.

The point here is not that it is implausible, or unwarranted, to believe that I can share non-superficial features with someone to whom I am closely genetically related (largely in virtue of that close relation). We often share such features. And if you share those features and *know* you share those features then, indeed, that other person could potentially be a source of self-knowledge (although it is worth emphasizing again that the more complex or subtle the shared feature is, the less confident you should be that the precise ways in which the feature manifests in the other person are also how it manifests in you). The key thought is that you already have to know (or at least have a pretty good idea) that you share the relevant features. And to know that you need to already have substantially answered the question "What am I (like)?" Acquiring genetic knowledge, then, is not a particularly effective way of answering this identity question.

5. "Who am I like?"

But the mirror metaphor is not bunk. We just need to interpret it differently. Rather than seeing it as a metaphor for learning *what* one is like, we should see it as a metaphor for *who* one is like. When someone says "It was like looking in a mirror!" they are remarking on how similar the person they are looking at is to them, and this is the thing that fascinates. Consider the following two remarks by donor-conceived people, whom I'll call "Ron" and "Rachel":[33]

---

[33] I made up the first since the source is anonymous. The second is the name provided by the authors in Amanda J. Turner and Adrian Coyle, "What Does It Mean to Be a Donor Offspring?

Ron: I wasn't prepared for how radical meeting my bio father would be. I expected that perhaps I might understand myself better, but I had this really profound moment where I came home from my first meeting with my biological father and looked at myself in the mirror. It felt like my face was different, like I was actually seeing it for the first time.[34]

Rachel: I needed to know whose face I was looking at in the mirror—I needed to know who I was and how I came to be—it was a very primal and unrelenting force which propelled the search and it was inescapable and undeniable.[35]

Talk of mirrors—literal mirrors!—figures into both Ron's and Rachel's accounts of the significance of knowing who their donor is. But the significance does not seem to have to do with learning *what* they are, but more simply *who* they are like.

Consider Ron. It is possible that after meeting his genetic father Ron literally discovered—upon looking in a mirror again—that he had certain facial features he didn't realize he had. Perhaps features that previously were not salient to him became salient. What is more likely, however, is that certain features that he had always noticed took on a new significance in light of their resemblance to his genetic father. Those features, which Ron always knew he had, *now answered to someone*, so to speak. The same thought is even more evident in Rachel's statement that she "needed to know whose face I was looking at in the mirror." She knows it is her face! What she wants to know is *who else* has a face like hers.[36]

The Identity Experiences of Adults Conceived by Donor Insemination and the Implications for Counselling and Therapy," *Human Reproduction* 15, no. 9 (2000): 2041–51.

[34] We Are Donor Conceived, "Voices from the Offspring: Identity Formation," November 13, 2017, https://www.wearedonorconceived.com/personal-stories/voices-from-the-offspring-identity-formation/.
[35] Turner and Coyle, "What Does It Mean to Be a Donor Offspring?," 2046. We encountered this person in chapter 2 where I reported on how she recounts the effect of *the secret* on her life:

It [the withholding of information] created a "shroud of secrecy" and a "sense of shame" about something I could sense, but of what I had no real knowledge—I always had suspected something wasn't "kosher"—but didn't know what it was—there's no way my sense of self-esteem could not have been damaged by that experience.

It is important, I think, to bear this in mind when reading the very strong language she uses to describe her interest in knowing who her donor is.
[36] Although this is too simple an expression of the thought. I say a lot more about what this simple version of the thought might be getting at below.

This suggests that people are interested in *who* they are like not as a (limited) means for knowing *what* they are like, but rather because knowing who you are like is a basic part of determining your identity. We become interested in certain aspects of what we are like because those features are the ones that are related to *who* we are like. When James looked in the mirror and saw what he had *always* seen, it had a new relational significance: "I look like *him*." When Rachel looks in the mirror, at least some of the features she sees do not have that relational significance.

There is no doubt that people are interested in their resemblance to family members.[37] We can see this in the ubiquity of the "resemblance game": "You have my eyes, but your father's chin." "You look so much like your father! The spitting image!" We play the game with non-physical features too: "We are two peas in a pod: we both love to plan and organize." The point of this game isn't to gain self-knowledge—oftentimes both parties already know what they are like. The point, rather, is to emphasize *who* you are like: what you are like (in some respect) is the same as what some other person is like (in some respect). There is something about the fact of resemblance itself that seems to have significance for many people.[38]

It is easy to see how gaining genetic knowledge could help answer the question "Who am I like?" A child who bears no, or only a partial, genetic relation to his parents may well find himself with some features that other members of the family do not have. To the extent that this is an issue for the child it is *not* because they do not know themselves, that they are not sure *what* they are like. On the contrary, they know exactly what they are like and see that no one else in the family is like *that*.

Consider the story of Jorge, William, Carlos, and Wilber, two sets of identical twin brothers from Colombia. Due to a mix-up at the hospital shortly after their birth, they were raised as fraternal twins in different families.

---

[37] For discussion of how families with donor-conceived children navigate these choppy waters, see Gay Becker, Anneliese Butler, and Robert D. Nachtigall, "Resemblance Talk: A Challenge for Parents Whose Children Were Conceived with Donor Gametes in the US," *Social Science & Medicine* 61, no. 6 (2005): 1300–1309.

[38] Some evidence that donor-conceived people who want genetic knowledge are interested in the question "Who am I like?" more than the question "What am I like?" comes from Joanna E. Scheib, Alice Ruby, and Jean Benward, "Who Requests Their Sperm Donor's Identity? The First Ten Years of Information Releases to Adults with Open-Identity Donors," *Fertility and Sterility* 107, no. 2 (2017): 483–93. They found that among people who were conceived with an open donor and who requested information about their donor, by far the most common motivation for wanting genetic information "was based on the desire for more information—important enough that they were willing to put significant effort into obtaining their donor's identity. Most focused on wanting to know who he was as a person and what he looked like" (7).

Table 4.1 The mixed-up brothers of Bogota

The Mixed-Up Brothers of Bogota	Genetic brother pair 1	Genetic brother pair 2
Social brother pair 1	**Jorge**	Carlos
Social brother pair 2	William	**Wilber**

Source: Susan Dominus, "The Mixed-Up Brothers of Bogotá," *New York Times*, July 9, 2015, https://www.nytimes.com/2015/07/12/magazine/the-mixed-up-brothers-of-bogota.html.

The relations are mapped out in Table 4.1 (the boldface names indicate the brothers that were raised by their genetic parents).

As Susan Dominus describes it:

> That Carlos never looked like Jorge and Diana [his social mother] was obvious. His siblings shared their mother's more delicate frame, her high cheekbones, her eyes. Carlos was taller, solidly built, with a wider nose and a heavier brow. The contrast was not merely physical: Carlos had always felt like an outlier in his family, although he preferred to think of himself as independent. As a child, Carlos had no interest in joining the elaborate games of make believe that his mother and siblings played, the funny voices they each put on, playacting for hours. [. . .] He was the only one in his family who cared about fashion, and God knows he was the only one who could dance. Carlos and Jorge had always assumed that Carlos took after their father, but they did not know him well enough to be sure.[39]

Carlos knows what he is like: tall, solidly built, wide nose, heavy brow, independent, little interest in playacting or games, lots of interest in fashion, a good dancer. What he (and Jorge) did not know was *who* Carlos was like. Acquiring genetic knowledge could—and to a large extent *did*—tell them that. And it could do the same for many donor-conceived people.

What explains the interest in resemblance? Is there something about the fact of resemblance itself, or is the interest in resemblance a proxy for, or perhaps parasitic on, an interest in something else? Let's approach these

---

[39] Susan Dominus, "The Mixed-Up Brothers of Bogotá," *New York Times*, July 9, 2015, https://www.nytimes.com/2015/07/12/magazine/the-mixed-up-brothers-of-bogota.html.

questions by way of two others: Are there conditions under which people would lose their interest in resemblance? And if there are, would something remain that was still (and perhaps was always the thing) of interest?

To make these questions more tractable, let's focus on physical resemblance with respect to phenotypic traits that are largely insensitive to environmental influence, such as eye color. And now let's imagine a different way in which human reproduction could function. Consider Chance World. In Chance World genes play no special role in determining the phenotype of the resulting offspring. All children are equally likely to end up with any particular phenotypical trait. There is nothing about the genetic parents' particular genetic makeup that makes it more or less likely that the child will have certain phenotypical traits than others. Rather, the set of phenotypical traits the child ends up with is a matter of chance. Parents, in effect, create a featureless lump of clay, and chance determines what the resultant statue looks like. It is possible for a child to resemble her parents in Chance World. But if she does, it is just a coincidence. She is just as likely to resemble the person next door.

It is hard to know how we—if we were inhabitants of Chance World—would think of resemblance between genetic parents and their offspring. To the extent that people really did see resemblance as a matter of chance, I suspect they would not treat it as especially significant. It is true that in our world people point out resemblances between people who are not related (I've been told I look like John Kerry and Michael Phelps). But such resemblances aren't taken to have any real significance, suggesting that what interests us in the actual world is not the mere fact of resemblance, but rather something else.

What is that "something else"? I think there are two plausible answers. To address them, consider these two broad features of human reproduction:

1. The *schema*[40] for the phenotypic traits a person will have comes from the mixing of genetic material of two individuals (at least).[41]
2. The *elements (or contents) of the schema* are made up, as it were, of the content of the genetic parents' own schemas. The result is that there tends to be significant resemblance between the "structures" that result from the new schema and the originators' own schemas.

---

[40] People often talk of a genetic "blueprint," but such talk underplays the extent to which many, many phenotypical traits are sensitive to factors outside the gene. I prefer talk of a genetic "schema," which, I think, does not suggest that all the phenotypic details, so to speak, are already written into the genetic plan.

[41] In some cases, there might be three: an egg provider, a sperm provider, and a mitochondria provider. In principle there could be even more.

Some elements of a new schema are quite determinate and largely insensitive to environmental factors. Eye color, for example, is determinate in the schema (that one's eyes will be blue is given by the schema) and largely insensitive to environmental factors (how you are raised will not change your eye color). The same is true with respect to a large number of physical phenotypical traits, with the result that children tend to look like one, or both, of their genetic parents.

Things could have been different. Consider Very Different Schema World, where everyone has two sets of genetic schemas: the one that determines many of their own phenotypical traits and another, *very different* schema that is passed on if they reproduce—the "reproduction schema." The schemas of children—and so many of their phenotypical traits—are a function of the combination of their genetic parents' reproduction schemas.[42]

In Very Different Schema World, the first feature of human reproduction is present—the resulting child's schema is given to them by her genetic parents. But the second feature is not: the elements of the child's schema are not made up of the elements of the genetic parents' schema (beyond general features shared by almost all humans), and so children in Very Different Schema World do not resemble their genetic parents in the way that they tend to in our world.

Now consider another possibility. In First Six Months World people's phenotypes are extremely changeable. People are born with certain phenotypical features, but those features are highly unstable for the first six months of their life. Their permanent phenotypical features are determined by the phenotypes of the people who play a primary role in raising a child over its first six months of life. In other words, children take on the phenotypical features of their primary caregiver(s).

The first feature of human reproduction noted above is absent in First Six Months World. The schema for the phenotypic traits a person will ultimately have does not come from the mixing of genetic materials of two individuals. The second feature—resemblance between children and parents—will

---

[42] This thought experiment is similar to one from Neil Levy and Mianna Lotz, who imagine a "baby-making machine" which:

> allows its operator to construct a viable embryo, which is then implanted into a uterus (natural or artificial) and brought to term. The operator can select the genotype of the embryo, gene for gene. Thus she can build the baby from the ground up.

See Neil Levy and Mianna Lotz, "Reproductive Cloning and a (kind of) Genetic Fallacy," *Bioethics*, 19, no. 3 (2005): 232–250.

be present only to the extent that genetic parents tend to be social parents. But when a child is not raised by his genetic parents or their close genetic relatives, there will be no resemblance except by chance.

We now have three worlds to consider where children do not reliably resemble their genetic parents in virtue of being their genetic children: Chance World, First Six Months World, and Very Different Schema World. I have already suggested that in Chance World we would probably not be particularly interested in the fact that we resemble other people, at least not insofar as we internalize that such resemblance is just a matter of chance. I suspect our interest in resemblance in First Six Months World would be more or less as it is now. Now, it is true that *whom* we can resemble is different in First Six Months World than it is in our world. In our world, people tend to physically resemble their genetic parents. In First Six Months World, they would tend to resemble their social parents (genetic or not). But I don't see why that would change the nature of our interest in resemblance. It's just that the target of the interest would be different, namely social, rather than genetic, parents.

Why would we be interested in resemblance in First Six Months World but not in Chance World? The answer, I suspect, is that resemblance in First Six Months World is not a matter of, well, *chance*: children in First Six Months World resemble their (social) parents *because* of their social parents. The child in First Six Months World can truthfully say, "I look like you *because* of you. My schema both comes from you and is made up of elements of your schema." The child in Chance World cannot truthfully say this: if she looks like her parent(s) it is just a matter of dumb luck. This suggests that our interest in resemblance in the actual world is parasitic on the resemblance being the result of a mechanism that reliably produces resemblance between parents and children.[43]

Where does Very Different Schema World fit in? It might seem that what is true of Chance World is true of it as well: in both worlds there is no reliable resemblance between genetic parents and their children. But there is a crucial difference between the worlds. While in Chance World the child's phenotype

---

[43] Would a donor-conceived person who is the result of double donation be interested in obtaining genetic knowledge in First Six Months World? They might be. It is true that in First Six Months World, neither the question "What am I like?" nor "Who am I like?" could be answered for this child (at all) by acquiring genetic knowledge. But the question "How am I?" still can be. To the extent that a donor-conceived child engages with that question as part of the task of healthy identity formation and engages with it *via* the genetic route, then she will be interested in acquiring genetic knowledge. But overall, my guess is that people's interest in acquiring genetic knowledge in cases where one was not raised by one's genetic parents would be substantially diminished in First Six Months World.

is just a matter of chance, in Very Different Schema World it comes from the genetic parents. It just turns out that the child's schema is not reliably similar to their genetic parents'. So the child in Very Different Schema World can truthfully say a more limited version of what the child in First Six Months World can say. The latter can say: "I look like you because of you." The former can say: "I look like *this* because of you. My schema comes from you." The interest I am imagining here is related to the *kind* of person one is. The person in Very Different Schema World, I imagine, wants genetic knowledge because he is interested in knowing who made him the *kind* of person he is (at least in some ways), even if the people who made him the kind of person he is don't resemble him at all.[44]

We have, then, two interpretations of the question "Who am I like?" According to the first, the person who asks it is really asking something like "Who are the people that are like me and made me like I am (and so like them)?" According to the second, the person who asks it is really asking something like "Who made me like I am?" (without any interest in resemblance as such). There is a place in *our* world for genetic knowledge in answering both questions. Indeed, genetic knowledge is required for answering either interpretation of "Who am I like?" if someone is focused on phenotypic traits that are largely insensitive to environmental factors.

Now, on either interpretation of the question one might still wonder what value there is to the answers. Are they really worth knowing? Perhaps the answers amount to little more than a kind of trivia about biological relatedness ("Huh. Yeah, we really look alike. Biology is kind of cool!"). I think that is a legitimate way of thinking about the kinds of resemblance I've been talking about. But I don't think it is rationally mandated. Another kind of temperament may rationally see things differently. It is, in my view, remarkable that I—or indeed anyone—grew in another person as a result of a relatively small number of cells getting together, cells that carry with them a pretty substantial portion of the schema for the form of how I am embodied. It is, for me at least, wondrous that we all started from bits of other people, bits that carried in them the schema for so much of who we are and which borrow heavily from the schema of our progenitors. We are literally made from other people, not just in the sense that other people cause us to be (though that is true) but

---

[44] Here I disagree with Levy and Lotz who conjecture that people would generally not be interested in knowing the person who ran the baby-making machine that gave them their genotype (except, they note, in the case where someone used the machine to endow the resulting child with their own genotype). Levy and Lotz, "Reproductive Cloning and a (kind of) Genetic Fallacy", 245.

also in the sense that they constitute us. They make us, in no small way, what we are like. For someone who sees things this way, there is no mystery why someone might want to know their genetic progenitor as a way of answering the question "Who am I like?"

There is no doubt that some donor-conceived people see things this way, as do, I suspect, many people who are not donor-conceived. According to Rosanna Hertz and Margaret Nelson, two sociologists who studied cohorts of donor-conceived genetic half-siblings, when some donor-conceived people learn that they share some of their qualities with the donor, "they understand themselves better because *they can find a source*"[45] for those qualities. They want to know who made them the way they are (at least in some respects).

For someone who does not feel the sense of wonder I've tried to describe, what I've just said will ring as nothing more than a rhetorically dressed-up account of human reproduction. That's fine. I don't think the "wondrous" attitude is any more rationally mandated than the "biological trivia" attitude. What we have here, I think, is a kind of ground-level aspect-seeing. What moves one person may be a total bore to another. Neither is mistaken. We'll return to this pluralistic conclusion in a moment. The point I want to emphasize here is just that it is intelligible and, I would venture, fairly common for people to have the "wondrous" attitude (even if they wouldn't formulate it quite the way I do) and that it explains, at least in part, why knowing the source of what you are like matters to many donor-conceived people.

The skeptic might grant that the "wondrous" attitude is fairly common, but deny that it is rational on the grounds that it reflects a pervasive and unfounded genetic essentialism, i.e. the idea that what we are like is largely, and straightforwardly, a matter of our genetic endowment. They may point out that there is a tendency to oversimplify the story people tell themselves about why they are the way they are and that genetic relatedness often plays an outsize role in that story. By way of evidence for this line of thought, consider the following anecdotes from Hertz and Nelson's fieldwork. One of the people they interviewed was Debra,[46] a single mother who wanted a Jewish donor:

> She suggested she would be more comfortable with her child because that child would understand innuendo and humor and look like her; the Jewish "part" would enable a profound connection.

---

[45] Rosanna Hertz and Margaret K. Nelson, *Random Families: Genetic Strangers, Sperm Donor Siblings, and the Creation of New Kin* (New York: Oxford University Press, 2018), 45, emphasis added.
[46] These are not the actual names of the people Hertz and Nelson interviewed.

Debra: [. . .] If I say something with a Jewish innuendo, [if] you're from that side, you get the Jewish part. If I say something like that, she'll get it genetically.[47]

Or consider the story of Courtney, who read her donor's profile for the first time when she was 15:

His favorite sport is soccer and I had not known that. I play soccer too. He used to juggle, which is a really obscure talent that I had actually started. It's like this is very random. I thought this was funny—because his favorite type of music was alternative rock. We have similar music tastes. I believe if I had grown up during his time, we would have had similar taste in bands. I thought that was me . . . Dogs are also one of my favorite animals. He says, "Especially retriever-sized."[48]

In both of these stories, we see people crediting similarities (actual or desired) between a child and their genetic progenitor to a genetic mechanism that is non-existent. There is no gene—or set of genes—for getting Jewish humor (since there are no "Jewish" genes) or for liking alternative rock or for liking retriever-size dogs. If any traits are culturally mediated and transmitted, it is surely these three. And yet here we have two people who attribute them to a genetic mechanism, as though they are traits like eye color or the number of fingers a person has.

These are just two stories. But the skeptic may claim they reflect a mode of thought that is ubiquitous even if it is not universal: that our genetic endowment provides not a schema but a *blueprint*, a detailed set of instructions, which almost exhaustively dictates, from the moment of conception, what we will be like. The consequence is that people tend to both prioritize explanations of similarity and trait transmission that happen *via* genetic mechanisms, while also attributing shared traits to genetic mechanisms in a way that is unwarranted. And this, says the skeptic, raises the worry that the interest in knowing who one is like reflects nothing particularly valuable. It is, rather, the result of an unfounded genetic essentialism.[49]

---

[47] Hertz and Nelson, *Random Families*, 28–29.

[48] Hertz and Nelson, *Random Families*, 45–46.

[49] This essentialism is also manifest in how people tend to think about race in the context of assisted reproduction. As Camisha Russell puts it: "Race . . . tends to be treated by ART users and practitioners as a property that resides within human gametes (sperm or eggs) and that can be known by identifying the race of the person whence the gamete came. In other words, it seems to hold a sort of

This is a serious worry. It is part of a broader critique of the interest in genetic knowledge as nothing more than a function of a society that un-justifiably valorizes genetic relatedness. I consider this critique in detail in the next chapter. But there are two points I want to emphasize now. First, even though attempts to answer the question "Who am I like?" might often be wrapped up with problematic genetic essentialism, the interest in an-swering the question is nonetheless intelligible as part of the task of identity determination. Second, aiming to answer the question, at least in part, by acquiring genetic knowledge is legitimate even if explanations of similarity in terms of shared genes often go too far. This is simply because our genetic progenitors *are* a source—and not an insignificant one—of what we are like. Indeed, one theme in many accounts about donor-conceived people—and their families—seeing and interacting with their donor for the first time is the power of beholding striking similarities in features that *are* transmitted genetically. The skeptic is certainly right that people reach for genetics-based similarities where there are none to be found. But that observation does not undermine the rational intelligibility of wanting genetic knowledge as part of an answer to the question "Who am I like?"

Even so, there is a crucial lesson to be learned from the skeptic's challenge. The lesson comes from the obvious—but still often overlooked—point that not all phenotypical features of a person are largely insensitive to environ-mental influence. A person's genes will set constraints on what phenotypical features are possible for a person. But, as we've already noted, there is tre-mendous room for phenotypical variation within those constraints as a re-sult of a person's environment. And this opens other avenues for transmitting resemblance. As Charlotte Witt notes, we need to distinguish between

> [t]he heritability of a characteristic and the means by which it is herit-able. For a characteristic or trait to be heritable, there must be some way to ensure that offspring resemble their parents with respect to that fea-ture. One vehicle for heritability is the genetic mode of transmission, which coordinate[s] features with different genes or gene complexes in a

pseudogenetic status." Camisha A. Russell, *The Assisted Reproduction of Race* (Bloomington: Indiana University Press, 2018), 24. As Russell argues, the idea that race is a genetically heritable trait is an updated version of a pre-genetic "old metaphorical understanding" of heritability in terms of "blood" and retains much of its historical baggage. As she puts it, the advent of genetic science has not led us to "question our biological determinism; we simply make it genetic determinism" (127). For a great overview of the way in which the assisted reproduction industry in the United States participates in and encourages racial-essentialist thinking, see Russell, 45–46.

population. Another vehicle for transmission could be parents teaching their children to have a certain characteristic, like moodiness, thriftiness, or a wacky sense of humor.[50]

The upshot is that "[f]amily resemblances which are heritable via the gene are just one ingredient in a [person's] self-understanding; many important family resemblances are passed on in other ways."[51] To think otherwise is to be beholden to an implausible kind of genetic essentialism.

So, when we seek to answer the question "Who am I like?" (on either version of the question) we have a choice about where to look. The person who asks "Who am I like?" must have certain features in mind, however

---

[50] Witt, "Family Resemblances," 143. It's worth noting that Witt's use of the term "heritable" is an example of what Evelyn Fox Keller calls the "colloquial meaning" of the term, according to which "to be heritable is to be capable of being passed on through the generations, of being inherited." Keller, *The Mirage of a Space between Nature and Nurture*, 56. Talk of "heritability" in this context refers to the quality of some feature being heritable. We might ask about the heritability of musical talent, where we are wondering about the extent to which it is passed from one generation to the next. According to this understanding of the terms "heritable" and "heritability," we can sensibly ask "if my musical ability . . . is heritable" (59). Witt's point is that genetics, or more broadly biology, do not provide the only mechanism of how traits are passed from parents to children. The colloquial meaning of the term "heritability" departs significantly from the technical meaning of heritability in biology, which is a measure of "the degree of variation in a phenotypic trait in a population that is due to genetic variation between individuals in that population." "Heritability," Wikipedia, December 2, 2020, https://en.wikipedia.org/w/index.php?title=Heritability&oldid=991870300. Heritability in the technical sense is a statistical measure of the extent to which some phenotypic variant in a given population correlates with genetic differences. Crucially, heritability in the technical sense "neither depends on, nor implies anything about, the mechanisms of transmission (inheritance) from parent to offspring." Keller, *The Mirage of a Space between Nature and Nurture*, 61. Here is an illustrative example from Keller:

> Consider a trait that is known to be biologically inherited (i.e. repeated from generation to generation), such as, e.g., the number of hands an individual has. We would normally say that hand number is a heritable trait. But what is its technical heritability? Answer: zero, or very close to it. And the reason is that, while there is phenotypic variance in the human population (not everyone has two hands), this variance is almost entirely due to accidents, not genetics. The genetic variance relevant to hand number in the population at large is virtually nil. (61)

In other words, while it is true that the number of hands a person has is, in almost every case, a function of biology (i.e. is biologically inherited), the *variance* we see in hand number among people has, in almost all cases, nothing to do with genetics. So the technical heritability is "virtually nil." Examples can run the other way as well. That is, there can be phenotypic variance that is highly heritable (in the technical) sense, but not genetically determined in the sense that people's genes are the cause of the variance. For some good examples, see Ned Block, "Race, Genes, and IQ," *Boston Review*, May 5, 2017, http://bostonreview.net/science-nature-race/ned-block-race-genes-and-iq. One reason the distinction between colloquial and technical means of "heritability" is important to bear in mind is that you cannot make inferences about one based on the other. From the fact that the technical heritability of having two hands is "virtually nil" you clearly cannot conclude that genetics contributes virtually nothing to people having two hands. Measures of technical heritability have no application in the case of individuals and individual traits. It makes no sense to ask what the technical heritability of someone's musical ability is, for instance.

[51] Witt, "Family Resemblances," 143.

implicitly. She cannot have in mind the totality of all the ways she is. Rather, she is wondering (however implicitly), "Who am I like with respect to *these* features (my sense of humor, the color of my eyes, my thriftiness, the twist of my smile)?" And the features that she is interested in may not be (largely) genetically heritable features. Those features might largely be a matter of indifference to her.

The genetic chauvinist will need to say that this person is making a mistake. But it is hard to see what it is. Traits that are highly sensitive to upbringing are no less "real" than those transmitted through genes. And depending on the trait, they may be no less changeable, both because some socially sensitive traits will be very hard for a person to change—a sense of humor perhaps—and also because it can be relatively easy to change a lot of one's phenotypic traits that are largely insensitive to upbringing.[52] What reason, then, could there be to think that everyone should privilege the kind of resemblance that occurs through genetics rather than through other modes of transmitting shared features? The answer, quite simply, is that there isn't.

Thus even if genetic knowledge provides one way of answering the question "Who am I like?," it is certainly not the only way. Nor is it a necessary way. As with the other two identity questions, genetic knowledge *can*, *but need not*, figure into someone's search for the answer to "Who am I like?"

6. Determining our identities: an epistemic and agential task

I have argued that the task of healthy identity determination, of properly answering the question "Who am I?," consists of answering three questions: What am I (like)? Who am I like? and How am I? The first two questions have to do with the kind of person you are. The last has to do with your metaphysical identity.

Genetic knowledge is not particularly important for answering the question "What am I (like)?" since, apart from simple physical characteristics (which you could discern with the use of mirrors or photographs), using genetic knowledge to learn more about what you are like requires that you already have a pretty good handle on what you are like. Genetic knowledge,

---

[52] I have in mind here colored contact lenses. Dyeing your hair. Pinning back your ears. That kind of thing.

however, can play a key role in answering the questions "Who am I like?" and "How am I?" Pursuing the genetic route to answer these questions, then, provides one way of properly answering the question "Who am I?" It offers one route for determining one's identity in a healthy way. But as we've seen throughout, it is not the only route. One could provide satisfactory answers to the identity questions without genetic knowledge. There are choices to be made about how to go about answering the questions, and different routes will appeal to different people.

In fact, there are not only choices about how to answer the identity questions, but also about what questions one asks in the first place. Everyone is interested, to some extent, in the question "What am I like?" We cannot help but have some self-concept, some picture of how we look, how we behave, what we like and dislike, what our passions and talents are. Engaging with the question "What am I like?" is part of being a self-conscious creature. So there is no choice here (inasmuch as one is self-conscious!). But if what I said above is right, this identity question is precisely the one where the role for genetic knowledge is most limited.

The other two questions—"Who am I like?" and "How am I?"—do not seem unavoidable in the same way. Indeed, the question "How am I?" is almost entirely avoidable. It is true that someone who doesn't have *any* conception of how they came to be is missing some important information. But the problem here seems less about healthy identity determination and more about lacking some basic knowledge of human reproduction.

Lots of people *are* interested in the question "How am I?" For some, this takes the form of tracing their genetic lineage across generations. For others, it takes the form of an interest in (some) of the details of their conception.[53] But some people don't have any particular interest in this question. They are not struck by the extraordinary improbability of their coming to be. I think we should take this lack of interest at face value. What I mean by that is not just that we should accept that there are varying levels of interest in the question "How am I?" but that it is perfectly fine that this is the case. People who are not interested in the question are not making a mistake. They are just interested in different things. It turns out that the identity question where there is the strongest case for the view that a genetic answer is especially valuable,

---

[53] Velleman offers some reflections on why people are interested in the "How am I?" question (although he does not put things in quite those terms). Unsurprisingly, Velleman thinks that interest in answering the question—and answering it *via* the genetic route—is something like a universal human need. Velleman, "III. Love and Nonexistence," 262.

or somehow privileged, is the one that healthy identity formation does not require someone to engage with (much) at all.

We are now in a position to understand the sense in which we *determine* our identities. Sometimes when we talk of "determining" something, we have in mind a purely epistemic task: the answer is out there and our job is to figure it out. So, I might determine the temperature by looking at the thermometer outside my window. But there is a sense of "determine" that is not epistemic, but rather agential. When my spouse and I set out to determine who will pick up the kids from school, we are, in a sense, making up an answer that was not there to be found apart from our making it up.

The task of healthy identity determination is partly epistemic and partly agential. Not just *any* way of thinking of myself is healthy. My self-conception must be constrained by the facts. To that extent, healthy identity determination is an epistemic task. But what I hope is now clear is that it is not just an epistemic task. There are all kinds of options for how someone goes about answering the questions that lie at the heart of identity determination. First, there are options about which questions to focus on. Second, and more significantly, there are options about how to go about answering the questions. Crucially, the presence of these options is not just a function of our finite capacity to search for, and find, answers. That view of things assumes that what even counts as an answer—what is a relevant fact, what is a relevant feature of my individual identity—is settled. But it is not: there are choices about what counts as the relevant territory in the first place. Making these choices is the agential aspect of identity determination. Having settled on the territory, the epistemic task kicks in.

The metaphor of the mirror emphasizes the epistemic task. When we are looking for a literal mirror, we want to know how we look. That answer is "out there" waiting to be discovered, and the mirror will show it to you. You wonder: "How does my hair look?" There is an answer, and the mirror give it to you: it looks like this. The task of looking for, and in, an actual mirror is metaphorically expanded when it comes to identity determination. The goal is not to find out how one looks, but rather to see how the world gave rise to *me*, both in the sense of being a particular individual with a certain history and being an individual of a particular *kind*. But the metaphor suggests that the answer is there waiting for you to see it.

There is, no doubt, something to that idea. Genuine identity determination must be rooted in reality and so the task is, no doubt, partly epistemic. But whereas an actual mirror cedes basically no control to the looker when it comes to what is reflected back, the same is not true when it comes to the metaphorical mirror that helps with identity determination. For, as we have seen, there are all kinds of different things to look for and you cannot look for them all. Where you look for answers—indeed the *kind* of answers you are interested in in the first place—are partly a matter of choice. Identity determination is partly an agential task, a fact which is easily missed if we focus on the metaphor of the mirror, where one is a passive recipient of what is reflected back.[54]

I don't mean to suggest that the agential task always precedes the epistemic task. Someone might stumble on some fact about themselves that generates an interest in that very thing. In the Yoffe story above, a box of pictures in an attic generates an interest in the child's "other mother." More generally, the language of "choice" is not quite right. A combination of circumstance and personality might simply make it the case that a person's interest in answering the identity questions one way rather than another is not immediately in their control. Indeed, as I suggested in chapter 3, the fact that one is a donor-conceived person in a world of largely non-donor-conceived people may make it all but inevitable that a significant portion of donor-conceived people are interested in acquiring genetic knowledge.

But even so, there is room for agency here. One can work at "cultivating an attitude of indifference"[55] to one's genetic lineage in much the same way one can train oneself to take an interest in some things (jazz, for example) or lose an interest in other things (Facebook). "One possibility," Hallvard Lillehammer explains:

> is to develop a practical identity in full consciousness that there are gaps in certain core facts about one's genealogical origins, as someone who does not care (or does not care very much) about certain facts about the exact nature of his biological lineage. To put it differently: one type of person that you can become is someone who does not care (or care that much) where

---

[54] There's a way in which the mirror metaphor is unintentionally apt. Looking in an actual mirror can effectively answer particular kinds of questions (e.g. "What does my hair look like?"), but one needn't ask those questions in the first place. Having settled on a particular question that is answered by looking in a mirror, one goes searching for a mirror. But one might not have asked a question that can be answered by looking in a mirror.

The mirror is akin to one path of identity determination. If you ask certain kinds of questions, you'll go down a particular path of identity determination that requires a "mirror." But if you ask other questions, you might never need a "mirror" at all.

[55] Lillehammer, "Who Cares Where You Come From?," 106.

you come from; who your biological parents are; the home town of your paternal grandparents; that you are one of your biological father's five hundred donor children, or that you were biologically constituted by a mixture of leftovers on a dish.[56]

The fact that healthy identity determination is partly an agential task, that there are choice points along the route for how go about determining one's identity, provides support for the empirical finding from chapter 3, that not all donor-conceived people care about acquiring genetic knowledge. If the account of identity determination I have given in this chapter is right, then it makes perfect sense that some donor-conceived people, as well many non-donor-conceived people, have no particular interest in having genetic knowledge. There are all kinds of ways to healthily determine one's identity other than the genetic route. People who pursue, or emphasize, non-genetic modes of identity determination are not self-deceived, or acting in bad faith, or making the best of a bad situation. It is simply that their interests, their proclivities, lie elsewhere and so send them down a different, but equally worthy, path of identity determination.

Advocates of the Profound Prudential Good view mistake one path for healthy identity determination as the *only* path or, at least, as the major superhighway. They are genetic chauvinists. But we should be genetic pluralists. Being a pluralist on this matter, however, involves acknowledging that the genetic route is a distinctively valuable path. The value of focusing on a fact like "I look like you *because* of you" is different from the value of focusing on a fact like "We came together because you chose me," even though both are instantiations of the common value of healthy identity determination. In other words, the genetic path is not fungible with respect to other paths. But then neither are the other paths fungible with respect to the genetic path. Pursuing the genetic route relates to the overarching task of identity formation as playing music relates to the task of artistic engagement. It has a distinct value, but one is not thereby impoverished for not engaging with it.[57]

---

[56] Lillehammer, "Who Cares Where You Come From?," 106.
[57] Lillehammer, "Who Cares Where You Come From?," 106.

7. Conclusion: the Significant Interest view is not a sideshow

We can now see why the Significant Interest view is not a sideshow. The sideshow worry, recall, stemmed from the fact that the Significant Interest view appeals to the idea that a donor-conceived person's interest in genetic knowledge is worthwhile. This led to the objection that the *real* argument for why intended parents should use an open donor should go directly through claims about the value of genetic knowledge and not through a claim about the likelihood of donor-conceived people being subjectively interested in genetic knowledge (which is a mere sideshow).

The Sideshow objection is right in one way. The Significant Interest view needs to show that people's interest in acquiring genetic knowledge is not worthless. But having done that, we can now see why the sideshow worry is ultimately misplaced. Because genetic knowledge has *optional* prudential value, a direct appeal to its value won't straightforwardly get us to the conclusion that intended parents have a weighty reason to use an open donor. After all, lots of things have optional prudential value—consider, once again, music and painting—and yet it is hardly clear, to put it mildly, that parents have a weighty reason to make as many optional prudential goods available to their children as possible. I don't mean to suggest that there *couldn't* be a strong argument for this (strong) view. But even if there is, the argument for the view that intended parents should use an open donor *still* won't depend on a direct appeal to the value of genetic knowledge, but rather on a contentious—and in my view implausible—claim about the obligation of parents to maximize options for their children.

The argument behind the Significant Interest view is considerably easier to make since it depends on the simple thought that if intended parents can be confident *in advance* that their child will have a worthwhile significant interest in something, then they have a weighty reason to help their child satisfy that interest. It is true that if the interest were in something profoundly prudentially valuable, then the fact that the child is actually interested in it wouldn't bear much weight. But genetic knowledge doesn't have that kind of value.

As result, we cannot jettison the psychological point about donor-conceived people's foreseeable interest in acquiring genetic knowledge in favor of a direct appeal to the value of genetic knowledge. The problem with denying a donor-conceived person genetic knowledge is not that they are being deprived of something that is crucial for well-being as such. It is, rather, that they are intentionally being deprived of something that has optional prudential value *and* which we know in advance they are likely be strongly interested in having.

But even if my account of the value of genetic knowledge is plausible, indeed even if it is right, it does not on its own show that the interest that donor-conceived people tend to have in genetic knowledge is not morally problematic. It could turn out that even if genetic knowledge is valuable in the way I've claimed it is, the fact that donor-conceived people tend to be interested in it is a function of bionormative prejudice. If that is true, then the Significant Interest view is still in trouble. Considering, and responding to, the bionormative prejudice objection is the task of the next chapter.

5

The Bionormative Prejudice

I have never met my donor "father," and I have no desire to do so. I do not see this lack of contact with my biological father as something missing in my life, and I have no hurt at the fact of my creation. What does cause me hurt, however, is the idea, constantly repeated . . . that there must be something wrong with your life if you do not know your biological father. My whole life I have been subjected to the shocked responses of people who—on learning that I don't know my donor—could not understand how I could be comfortable with this and believed I must be harboring hurt about it.
—Anonymous blog post on *Anonymous Us*, 2011

The "search for identity" does not exist in a vacuum.
—Katherine O'Donovan, *Birthrights: Law and Ethics at the Beginnings of Life*, 2003

Many donor-conceived people develop a significant interest in gaining genetic knowledge. This is not surprising. And because it is not surprising, someone conceiving a child with donated gametes has a weighty reason to use an open donor since doing so will put their future child in a good position to fulfill the significant interest she is likely to have. That, in a nutshell, is the Significant Interest view.

The heart of the view depends on the simple idea that, in general, parents should help their children achieve the things that matter to them (the children). But what if what matters to the child, what interests her, *isn't worth caring about*? The Significant Interest view indirectly answers this question in its appeal to the Well-Being Principle:

Well-being and significant interests: How well your life goes for you is partly (if not largely) a function of how successful you are in satisfying your

Conceiving People. Daniel Groll, Oxford University Press. © Oxford University Press 2021.
DOI: 10.1093/oso/9780190063054.003.0005

non-instrumental, significant, *worthwhile* interests. If you satisfy a non-instrumental, significant, worthwhile interest, then, to that extent, your life goes better for you.

Recall that by "worthwhile" I mean something fairly minimal: the interest is neither trivial nor morally problematic. The argument from chapter 4 is enough to show that people's interest in genetic knowledge is not trivial. But it might nonetheless be morally problematic. This is the objection I consider in this chapter.

Now the Well-Being Principle only says that satisfying your worthwhile significant interests is good for you. It doesn't say that satisfying your morally problematic significant interests isn't *also* good for you. But I have taken for granted that the interest in genetic knowledge *is* worthwhile. Moreover, it is hardly clear—to put it mildly—that parents have a weighty reason to help their children satisfy their morally problematic significant interests, even if doing so is good for their child. So, if the interest in genetic knowledge is morally problematic, then the Significant Interest view is in trouble.

Properly understood, however, the claim that people's interest in genetic knowledge is morally problematic has a lot of force. One goal of this chapter is to show why that is. But the second goal of the chapter is to show that the sense in which it is plausible does not, in fact, threaten the Significant Interest view.

I start by distinguishing between two kinds of morally problematic interests, what I call *baldly immoral interests* and *insidiously morally problematic interests*. I then introduce what Charlotte Witt calls the "bionormative conception of the family"[1] and show why it is plausible that an interest in genetic knowledge is a function of it. After that, I consider the view that the bionormative conception of the family evinces a bionormative *prejudice* that would, in turn, make the interest in genetic knowledge insidiously morally problematic. I consider, but ultimately reject three responses to this challenge before turning to a fourth, and my preferred, response to the Bionormativity objection.

---

[1] Charlotte Witt, "Family, Self and Society: A Critique of the Bionormative Conception of the Family," in *Family-Making: Contemporary Ethical Challenges*, ed. Carolyn MacLeod and Françoise Baylis (New York: Oxford University Press, 2014), 49.

1. Two kinds of morally problematic interests

1.1. Baldly immoral interests

What makes an interest morally problematic? Suppose Annie has a serious interest in torturing small animals. To call this interest "morally problematic" seems to understate things considerably. Annie's interest is baldly immoral. It is pretty easy to tell baldly immoral interests when we see them. They are *baldly* immoral, after all. But it is worth saying something about their features as preparation for thinking about whether an interest in genetic knowledge is morally problematic.

1. Its content is baldly immoral. It is an interest in (doing) something that is very obviously wrong. What makes it obviously wrong is that it involves intentionally and substantially harming or disrespecting something with moral status (in an unjustifiable way).
2. In general it is not reasonable for people to have baldly immoral interests. This is not to say that we cannot understand why they have them. It is not hard to imagine story that would make sense of Annie's love of torturing small animals. Nonetheless, people in general shouldn't have baldly immoral interests. If they can abandon them, then they should.
3. Acting on a baldly immoral interest is usually blameworthy.
4. Having a baldly immoral interest is usually partly constitutive of having a bad character. It reflects poorly on Annie as a person that she is interested in torturing small animals (if nothing else, it shows a real insensitivity to the suffering of sentient creatures).

Suppose Annie's parents could see in advance that Annie was likely to develop a serious interest in torturing small animals. We would not think they must prepare the ground for her to successfully pursue that interest! Indeed, we would think they should do what they can to prevent her from developing the interest in the first place. But even if they couldn't do that, even if it turned out that Annie's interest in torturing small animals was largely immune to parental influence, we probably don't think that her parents have a weighty reason, let alone a decisive one, to put Annie in a position to succeed at fulfilling her interest in torturing small animals. Indeed, her parents may have decisive reason to work to frustrate the interest (even if they cannot rid her of it).

If donor-conceived people's interest in genetic knowledge is baldly immoral, then the Significant Interest view won't go through (just as the torturing small animals version of the view wouldn't go through). But the interest in genetic knowledge is not baldly immoral. It certainly doesn't have baldly immoral content, and not just in the sense that the content is bad but not *that* bad. The content doesn't involve intentionally and substantially harming or disrespecting anyone (or anything). Moreover, I doubt most people think anyone acting on the interest in genetic knowledge should be blamed or that having the interest makes them a bad person. We tend to think it is a perfectly reasonable interest to have.

But now we might well wonder: If it has none of the marks of a baldly immoral interest, why think that it is morally problematic?

1.2. Insidiously morally problematic interests

Imagine that Marlena, a 15-year-old girl, has a significant interest in having a nose job because, she says, her nose is just "too big" and no one will find her attractive. Or imagine that Otis, a 16-year-old boy, has a significant interest in "bulking up" because otherwise, everyone will think he is wimpy.[2] What should we make of these highly gendered interests?

Imagine you were Marlena's parents and she positively begged you for a nose job. Assuming that cost was not an issue, would you accede? Why isn't the answer *obviously* "yes"? Here is something your child is really interested in. And she may well be right that she will feel better, perhaps even be happier, with a "new" nose. Moreover, it is not clear at all that anyone is harmed if she gets a nose job. Put this way, her interest doesn't look so different from a child's keen interest in taking up the piano or joining the swim team. Assuming it doesn't impose an outsize burden, it seems clear that parents should help her meet the interest.

But we *wouldn't* feel that way about the nose job if we were Marlena's parents.[3] Part of the reason, no doubt, is that we're talking about surgery and

---

[2] I don't mean to suggest that gendered interests are entirely symmetrical. As Marilyn Frye has argued, the gendered "restraints" that govern men are imposed by men and generally for the benefit of men. The gendered restraints that govern women are *also* imposed by men and generally for the benefit of men. Marilyn Frye, *The Politics of Reality: Essays in Feminist Theory* (Berkeley, CA: Crossing Press, 1983), 14.

[3] I think this is particularly clear if we switch the example to something like breast-augmentation surgery, but I favor the subtler nose-job example. The reason is that if the interest in genetic knowledge is morally problematic, it is fairly subtly morally problematic. It doesn't wear its problematic

all the risks and unpleasantness that it entails. But surely that is only part of the explanation. For it seems a pity that Marlena has the interest in having a "prettier" nose in the first place. We rightly resent that we live in a society that valorizes women's appearance alongside a very narrow conception of beauty. More generally, we rightly lament the interests that people have that are a function of a problematic social context. Gendered interests, like those of Otis and Marlena, are prime examples. They result from deeply problematic societal structures and attitudes.

Other examples abound. Consider, for example, the interest that a Black person in the United States has in behaving in a so-called respectful or deferential way around law enforcement; or the interest that a gay person living in a rural, conservative part of the United States might have in behaving a certain way at the local bar. Giving in to the interest feels like acceding to something not only unfair, but also demeaning.

But here's the thing: we recognize not only the significance of these kinds of interests in people's lives, but also the genuine importance of the interests being met. The importance is genuine in the sense that having the interest, and having it satisfied, is very likely to benefit, or more modestly, prevent harm to, the interest-holder (beyond the possible psychological benefit of the interest being met). A Black person who conforms to certain expectations about behavior around law enforcement could well save his own life. To not give in to the interest is not a live option, given the danger it puts the interest holder in. Unlike with baldly immoral interests, we do not merely *understand* why people have interests like these (in the way that we can understand how Annie came to love torturing small animals). We also think that it is *reasonable* for the person to have them. When we tally up the balance of reasons for, and against, having the interest we either see (a) that the scale tilts (sometimes rather obviously) toward having the interest or at least (b) that someone could reasonably think it does. Indeed, being the parents of a Black child in the United States or a gay child in certain communities often involves actively inculcating the interests mentioned above in your child for their own benefit:

> To be Black in America is to spend a lot of time talking about how to avoid death. Conversations with my sons go something like this:

nature clearly on its sleeve (if it is problematic). The nose-job example is like that too, at least compared to the breast-augmentation example.

"Keep your hands within your car when (not if) a white police officer pulls you over."

"Don't pull out your cellphone or your wallet carelessly, because around white people those things magically become weapons."

"Don't blast your music in your car, as this can be offensive to whites within earshot."

"Don't sit in a Starbucks and have to use the restroom."

"Don't take a nap at your university unless you are in *your room*."

Hell, I even tell them not to feel too comfortable while in their own home.[4]

These interests are perfectly rational.[5] And yet, what a pity and injustice that this is so. What a shame that someone who is Black needs to watch their behavior in certain contexts so as to avoid suffering substantial harm. Crucially, what makes it a shame is not that the world just happens to be arranged so as to make having the interests in question reasonable. Rather it is the fact that the world is arranged that way *as a result* of racial prejudice, both individual and systemic.[6] The context that makes having the interests in question reasonable is deeply morally problematic. So while we understand why someone has the interest, indeed while it is reasonable to have the interest, we think overall that it would best if there were *no need* to have the interest. The interest, we might say, is a function of a morally problematic milieu, one that should be different than it is and thereby obviate the need for the interest.

Does that make the interest itself morally problematic? No. Someone who has a significant interest in fighting institutional racism, for example, has an interest that is a function of morally problematic circumstances. But the interest itself is obviously not morally problematic—quite the contrary. So if we want to capture the thought that there is something morally problematic with the kind of interests I mentioned above, but not with an interest in fighting

---

[4] George Yancy, "Opinion: Ahmaud Arbery and the Ghosts of Lynchings Past," *New York Times*, May 12, 2020, https://www.nytimes.com/2020/05/12/opinion/ahmaud-arbery-georgia-lynching.html.

[5] Sally Haslanger: "The current racial structure (and gender structure) in the United States is morally problematic and I seek ways to undermine it, and yet I also believe that it would be wrong not to teach my children how to situate themselves as Black (and gendered) within that structure." Sally Haslanger, "Family, Ancestry, and Self," in *Resisting Reality: Social Construction and Social Critique* (New York: Oxford University Press, 2012), 167.

[6] The dynamic I'm describing here is what Marilyn Frye famously described as a "double bind" wherein "options are reduced to a very few and all of them expose one to penalty, censure or deprivation." Frye, *The Politics of Reality*, 2.

institutional racism, it is not enough to say that the former is a function of a morally problematic milieu (since the latter is too). So, what is the difference?

Let's start with the gendered interests. The interest in conforming to gender norms mirrors, or *reflects*, the problematic attitudes that give rise to it. It is it-self an expression of those problematic attitudes. I'll call it a *reflective interest*.

The interest in fighting institutional racism is not a reflective interest: it does not reflect back the problematic attitudes that gave rise to it. On the con-trary, it aims to combat those very attitudes. It is an example of what I will call an *oppositional interest*.

The interest in behaving a certain way around police complicates this pic-ture. Like the gendered interests we've looked it, it mirrors the morally prob-lematic attitudes that give rise to it in the first place. It is, then, a reflective interest. But it is plausibly importantly different from the gendered interests we have been looking at. For consider the likely attitude of the person who has an interest in being deferential to police officers to that very interest. In all likelihood, he recognizes it for what it is: an unfortunate tool to avoid harm. We can easily imagine him thinking, "I need to be especially deferential in my interactions with police. That is bullshit, but that is the world I am in." In other words, he holds the interest grudgingly.[7] He simultaneously recognizes that it would be best if there were no need for him to have the interest at all, but that having (and satisfying) it is crucial given the way the world is.[8]

Interests like those of Marlena and Otis are often not like this. They are not held grudgingly. Rather the interest holder endorses the content. It takes up residence in their minds.[9] The destructive potential of such internalization is powerfully articulated by James Baldwin in his letter to his nephew, where he says of his father, "He had a terrible life; he was defeated long before he died because, at the bottom of his heart, he really believed what white people said about him."[10] It is easy to imagine that Marlena really thinks that people with smaller noses are more beautiful and that Otis really thinks that being strong (in some traditional sense) is how a man ought to be. They have internalized the problematic norms embedded in the problematic interest. As Frye puts it:

---

[7] William Edward Burghardt Du Bois, *The Souls of Black Folk* (New York: Oxford University Press, 2008), 45.

[8] The "double bind," we might say, is fully in view for him.

[9] To paraphrase a memorable line from Sandra Lee Bartky, *Femininity and Domination: Studies in the Phenomenology of Oppression* (New York: Routledge, 2015), 2.

[10] James Baldwin, *The Fire Next Time* (New York: Knopf Doubleday, 2013), 4.

Many of the restrictions and limitations we live with are more or less internalized and self-monitored, and are part of our adaptations to the requirements and expectations imposed by the needs and tastes and tyrannies of others.[11]

We have in view, then, the kind of interests I am interested in. Internalized reflective interests are, as I shall put it, *insidiously morally problematic*. Unlike baldly immoral interests, insidiously morally problematic interests aren't about intentionally and substantially harming others in an unjustifiable way.[12] Moreover, insidiously morally problematic interests are not unreasonable to have. Indeed they can be perfectly rational responses to oppressive circumstances. Consequently, acting on an insidiously morally problematic interest is not apt to be blameworthy. But these interests are, nonetheless, morally problematic inasmuch as they reflect and endorse morally problematic features of the society that gave rise to them. As Sandra Bartky puts it, they "arise from oppressive intersubjective relationships and . . . tend at the same time to reproduce and reaffirm those very relationships."[13]

2. The Bionormativity objection

So we have a contrast between baldly immoral interests and insidiously morally problematic interests. The distinction is neither sharp nor exhaustive.

---

[11] Frye, *The Politics of Reality*, 13. Paul Benson likewise distinguishes between interests generated by merely "coercive pressures," by which he means pressures that the subject (rightly) experiences as coercive, and "primary" interests that result from the subject of the coercive pressure *internalizing* the problematic norms and values. Paul Benson, "Autonomy and Oppressive Socialization," *Social Theory and Practice* 17, no. 3 (1991): 387–88.

[12] If there is harm done to others by someone having, and acting on, an insidiously morally problematic interest, it is highly diffuse.

[13] Bartky, *Femininity and Domination*, 2. A similar point holds for even grudgingly held morally problematic interests, which also serve to entrench morally problematic norms and structures. A person of color who is especially deferential to police, for example, is (totally understandably and reasonably) further entrenching expectations—and the attendant attitudes—about what appropriately interacting with law enforcement looks like for a person of color. To that extent, even grudgingly held morally problematic interests are insidiously morally problematic. But it certainly matters, morally speaking, that they are held grudgingly. On the one hand, grudgingly held morally problematic interests alienate the interest holder from himself. He has an interest in doing something that he realizes debases or disrespects himself. On the other hand, they do not penetrate to the soul, so to speak, of the interest holder. The infection is, in a way, at the surface of the person's character. They also allow for competing significant interests to be coherently held. One can coherently have a significant interest in, for example, being especially deferential to police while at the same time having a significant interest in fighting against a system that makes it reasonable for a person of color to have an interest in being especially deferential to law enforcement.

Some interests that are intuitively morally problematic, but not baldly immoral, will not be the result of oppression. And some interests that are baldly immoral will be the result of oppression. But we needn't worry about these subtleties. Why? Because the claim we are interested in is that genetic knowledge isn't worthwhile in a paradigmatic way, at least according to the paradigm I articulated above.

We are now in position to see why the idea that an interest in genetic knowledge is morally problematic is not as implausible as it might have initially seemed to some. The best version of the view maintains that donor-conceived people's interest in genetic knowledge is insidiously morally problematic. We can understand why people have the interest. Indeed, we might well think it is reasonable that they do *given the society we live in*, i.e. a society that is shot through with bionormativity. Just what this means is something we'll get to in a second, but the general claim is clear enough. Our society privileges family forms that are structured around genetic relatedness. People who are raised in contexts where they are cut off from their genetic progenitors are thought to be missing something. It is no surprise, then, that such a person growing up in such a society would come to see herself as missing something and so develop a significant interest in finding it. The interest has the hallmarks of an insidiously morally problematic interest. It is a function of oppression, reflects that oppression, and further entrenches the oppression.

2.1. The bionormative conception of the family

What does it mean to say that our society is shot through with bionormativity? To answer that question, consider three cultural vignettes. The first is the (extremely catchy and awesome) song *Hey Sister!* by Walter Martin. Here are some of the words:

Brother: Hey, sister.
Sister (spoken): Yeah?
Brother: Something in the way you look looks just like me.
Sister (spoken): Well that kinda makes sense, I mean I *am* your sister.
Brother: And something in the way you talk sounds just like Aunt Marie.
Sister (spoken): Yeah, I could see that.
Brother: And Grandma looks just like Pop.
Sister (spoken): It's true, isn't it?

Brother: And Mamma looks just like Cousin Bob. We should put 'em all together and call it a family.

Both: There's a tiny little bit of me in you and a tiny little bit of you in me. Your hair is messy and your eyes are blue. I guess we fell out of the same tree. Coincidentally.

Sister: Hey, brother.

Brother (spoken): Uh huh?

Sister: You're pretty funny—you must have got that from me.

Brother (spoken): Uh, I'm not sure if that's technically possible. Is it actually?

Sister: And you sing kinda funny—you must have got that from Grandaddy.

Brother (spoken): What exactly do you mean by that?

Sister: And Uncle Jack's got Mommy's laugh.

Brother (spoken): Yeah, that's true.

Sister: And Uncle Jim's got Dad's old mustache.

Brother (spoken): Yeah, that's right.

Sister: We should put 'em all together and call it a family.[14]

The second cultural vignette is, simply, a sign I saw outside a liquor store in Scotland on Mothering Sunday: "She birthed you. So buy her a beer!" The final vignette is a collection of nearly identical stories:

1. The philosopher Hallvard Lillehammer recounts that when he was a young child, he was sent to school in a small town. On the first day of school, upon arriving in the playground, an older boy came up to him and asked, right off, "Who is *your* father?"[15]

2. The mother of a donor-conceived child recounts, "I think the first time it ever actually came up in a conversation he was about 3 and a half, maybe 3, and a friend of his . . . asked him 'where's your dad, have you got a dad?' And I could see him thinking, 'Hold on a second, I don't.' "[16]

3. Maybell Murphy-Sylla, a donor-conceived eighth-grader from California, writes: "I've known my whole life that I'm a sperm donor child. [. . .] I considered it completely normal. When I was about eight, I started to hear otherwise. I received many apologies from my peers

---

[14] Walter Martin, *Hey Sister* (New York: Family Jukebox, 2014).

[15] Thanks to Hallvard for letting me use this story.

[16] Tabitha Freeman et al., "Disclosure of Sperm Donation: A Comparison between Solo Mother and Two-Parent Families with Identifiable Donors," *Reproductive Biomedicine Online* 33, no. 5 (2016): 597.

when I told them that I didn't have a dad. Even my closest friend told me that she felt bad for me. I was asked if I would call the sperm donor 'dad' when I turned 18 and met him."[17]

These three vignettes—which could be replaced by countless others—evince a particular conception of what families are like: families consist of children, mothers, and fathers; the children are the genetic product of the mother and father and, as we might put it, the gestational product of their mother; the genetic relations within families explain similarities between family members (both immediate and more distant) and are what makes a family *a family*: "We should put 'em all together and call it a family." Or as David Schneider puts it in *American Kinship*:

> The blood relationship, as it is defined in American kinship, is formulated in concrete, biogenetic terms. Conception follows from a single act of sexual intercourse between a man, as genitor, and a woman, as genitrix. At conception, one-half of the biogenetic substance of which the child is made is contributed by the genitrix, and one-half by the genitor.[18]

This conception of the family—Schneider calls it the "biogenetic" conception of kinship,[19] Witt the "bionormative conception of the family,"[20] and Haslanger "*'the natural nuclear family'* schema"[21]—is not meant to capture what all families are actually like. Everyone knows that there are single-parent families, families with two dads, families with two moms, families with children who are not genetically related to both parents, etc.[22] Instead,

[17] Maybell Murphy-Sylla, "Sperm Donor Kid," KQED, February 26, 2020, https://www.kqed.org/perspectives/201601139597/sperm-donor-kid. Thanks to Alice MacLachlan for sending this story my way. As Hertz and Nelson point out, "For those in single-mother or two-mother families, interactions with other children raise questions about the absent 'father.' Children are left on their own to find an explanation for a missing parent." Rosanna Hertz and Margaret K. Nelson, *Random Families: Genetic Strangers, Sperm Donor Siblings, and the Creation of New Kin* (New York: Oxford University Press, 2018), 35–36.

[18] David M. Schneider, *American Kinship: A Cultural Account* (Chicago: University of Chicago Press, 2014), 23.

[19] Schneider, *American Kinship*, 21.

[20] Witt, "Family, Self and Society," 49.

[21] Haslanger, "Family, Ancestry, and Self," 179.

[22] Indeed, the bionormative family does not make up even half of families in the United States (although they do make up the plurality). Gretchen Livingston, "Fewer Than Half of US Kids Live in 'Traditional' Family," *Pew Research Center* (blog), December 22, 2014, https://www.pewresearch.org/fact-tank/2014/12/22/less-than-half-of-u-s-kids-today-live-in-a-traditional-family/.

the bionormative conception of the family expresses—if only implicitly—a view about what families *should* be:

> In our culture, according to the standard view of the family, there must be a genetic tie among its members, even though the parents in a family are normally not biologically related to one another. For us, therefore, what is meant by describing the family as a biological unit is that in the *ideal* families the children are biologically, or genetically, related to their parents.[23]

The upshot, according to Witt, is that "[f]amilies with children who are not genetically related to both their parents are not [considered] the gold standard or Platonic form of the family,"[24] and that "families formed via biological reproduction (in which there is a genetic relationship between parents and children) are, *for that reason*, [considered] superior to families formed in other ways."[25] The bionormative conception of the family can plausibly be seen as manifesting the kind of oppression that Iris Marion Young calls "cultural imperialism," which involves "the universalization of a dominant group's experience and culture, and its establishment as the norm."[26]

The choice to conceive children with donated gametes, particularly when combined with a reluctance to disclose to the child that she is donor-conceived, can be seen as reflecting the bionormative conception of the family inasmuch as it is an attempt to hew as closely as possible to the ideal of the bionormative family. "There is," Cahn says, "an attempt to replicate their 'as if' family."[27] It is no surprise why. Gamete conception takes place in a cultural context where biogenetic relationships are central, almost "mythical."[28] "When people enter the donor world," Cahn notes, "they are looking for children. And, almost always, they are hoping for children who will be

---

[23] Charlotte Witt, "Family Resemblances: Adoption, Personal Identity, and Genetic Essentialism," in *Adoption Matters: Philosophical and Feminist Essays*, ed. Sally Haslanger and Charlotte Witt (Ithaca, NY: Cornell University Press, 2005), 135.

[24] Witt, "Family, Self and Society," 49.

[25] Witt, "Family, Self and Society," 50.

[26] Iris Marion Young, *Justice and the Politics of Difference* (Princeton, NJ: Princeton University Press, 2011), 59. Young gets the term, and the general idea, from Maria C. Lugones and Elizabeth V. Spelman, "Have We Got a Theory for You! Feminist Theory, Cultural Imperialism and the Demand for 'the Woman's Voice,'" in *Women's Studies International Forum*, vol. 6 (Elsevier, 1983), 573–81.

[27] Naomi R. Cahn, *The New Kinship: Constructing Donor-Conceived Families* (New York: NYU Press, 2013), 54.

Cahn, *The New Kinship*, 54.

[28] Cahn, *The New Kinship*, 49. Cahn's invocation of the "mythical" status of biogenetic ties comes from David Schneider's *American Kinship*.

genetically related to them or to their partner."[29] Moreover, the choice of a particular donor often evinces a commitment to the importance of genetics for family formation:

> There are complex motivations with respect to choosing a donor, but [with couples] they often center on replicating the genetic makeup of the nonbiological parent and on ensuring that offspring are genetically related to one parent and to any potential siblings.[30]

Overall, the focus on the genetic connection that is simultaneously present and absent with donor conception promotes, "rather than challenge[s], the privileging and prioritizing of genetic ties."[31]

If all this is correct, it is easy to see why donor-conceived people are likely to develop an interest in genetic knowledge. Even if, as I argued in chapter 4, identity determination is partly agential—even if, that is, it is partly a matter of people choosing how to construct their identity—it is not an individualistic activity. Rather, it takes place in a context where other people and, more broadly, social structures foist their understanding of me (and you and everyone) on me (and you and everyone). In doing so, it makes some paths of identity determination more salient, more important, more seemingly necessary than others.[32]

The point about social structures is especially important to bear in mind. Bionormativity is not just the product of individual attitudes—like those on display in the cultural vignettes presented above—but also of institutional structures and practices that we all live with. To see this, consider three brief examples from the domains of medicine, education, and law.

Medical forms routinely ask for a patient's family medical history for Parent 1 and Parent 2, but do not distinguish between genetic family history and social family history. Suppose that the parent of a donor-conceived child is filling out this section of the forms for a doctor's visit. There is a history of alcoholism on the social, non-genetic side of the family. But there is a history

---

[29] Cahn, *The New Kinship*, 49. Velleman makes a similar point: "The reason for resorting to donated gametes in many cases, of course, is the desire of an adult to have a biologically related child, despite lacking a partner with whom he or she can conceive." J. David Velleman, "The Gift of Life," *Philosophy & Public Affairs* 36, no. 3 (2008): 371.

[30] Cahn, *The New Kinship*, 53.

[31] Cahn, *The New Kinship*, 54.

[32] As Leighton puts it: "[T]he diagnosis 'genealogical bewilderment' is itself generative of the very conditions of such suffering." Kimberly Leighton, "Addressing the Harms of Not Knowing One's Heredity: Lessons from Genealogical Bewilderment," *Adoption & Culture* 3 (2012): 65.

of thalassemia on the non-social, merely genetic side of the family (i.e. on the donor's side). How, then, to convey this "parental" medical history on the form? The point here is not that figuring out how to fill out the form presents some insurmountable obstacle. The point is that bionormativity is baked into the form itself, quite apart from whether anyone who works in the hospital or clinic has prejudicial bionormative attitudes.

The same is true when it comes to some educational practices. It is particularly on display when it comes to sex education, at least in large swaths of the United States. As Hertz and Nelson explain:

> When children are exposed to the "sex education" curriculum (usually in the fifth grade), even more questions emerge. The biology lessons explain that all kids are created from sperm and eggs; drawing on typical heteronormative schema, the lessons might also explain how the sperm and egg get together. Regardless of how much concrete information is provided, these conventional lessons do not include either reproductive technology (like in vitro fertilization) or the use of a donor.[33]

But even more mundane educational activities can evince and reinforce bionormativity. Carolyn McLeod's son failed an assignment about family history in grade school because he gave one-word answers (e.g. "Happy") to the questions "What did your grandfather feel like when you were born?" and "What did your mother feel like when you were born?" The teacher wanted more, but McLeod's son felt ill-equipped to say more because he was adopted as a toddler. He was not able (at the time) to ask his birth mother or his genetic grandfather how they felt. All he could do was speculate. He might have chosen to interpret "mother" and "grandfather" differently, but that wouldn't have helped since his adopted mother and grandfather didn't know of his existence when he was born. Perhaps he could have offered an answer that challenged the premise of the question. But these reactions miss the point. A question that was probably frictionless for most kids needed to be negotiated by McLeod's son precisely because his family does not fit the bionormative mold. The question threw his, and his family's, otherness into sharp relief.[34]

---

[33] Hertz and Nelson, *Random Families*, 36. I say more about this kind of education in chapter 8.

[34] This story comes from conversation and personal correspondence with Carolyn McLeod. Thank you to Carolyn for letting me use it here.

When it comes to law, Douglas NeJaime gives a series of examples of how non-bionormative families "struggle for parental recognition":[35]

> In Connecticut, a married different-sex couple had a child through surrogacy and raised the child together for fourteen years. When they divorced, the court deemed the mother, who had neither a gestational nor genetic connection to the child, a legal stranger to her child. In Florida, an unmarried same-sex couple used the same donor sperm to have four children, with each woman giving birth to two children. They raised the children together until their relationship ended several years later, at which point the court left each woman with parental rights only to her two biological children. In New Jersey, a male same-sex couple used a donor egg to have a child through a gestational surrogate. The court recognized the gestational surrogate, rather than the biological father's husband (and the child's primary caretaker), as the second parent.[36]

As with the cultural vignettes, these examples of bionormative social structures could be replaced with many others. The upshot of it all is that donor-conceived people experience an interpretive pressure to see their identity as bound up with their genetic origins. The quotation at the top of this chapter captures the pressure nicely. Something that had, perhaps, not been salient is *made* salient by other people's expectations. Ría Tabacco Mar captures this point when she writes about her daughter putting "I'm thankful for mommy and daddy" on a Thanksgiving Day craft, despite having two moms: "Kids reflect back what we show them."[37] And what we—as a society—show them every day, in ways large and small, is that the bionormative family is the ideal family. Ironically, attempts to disrupt that narrative can't help but draw attention to it. As Tabacco Mar explains, "stories featuring same-sex parents . . . tend to focus on the fact that having two moms or two dads

[35] Douglas NeJaime, "The Nature of Parenthood," *Yale Law Journal* 126, no. 8 (2017): 2260.

[36] NeJaime, "The Nature of Parenthood," 2265. The Connecticut example is Doe v. Doe, 710 A.2d 1297 (Conn. 1998). The Florida example is Russell v Pasik, 178 So. 3d 59–60 (Fla. Dist. Ct. App. 2015). The New Jersey example is A.G.R. v D.R.H, Unpub. LEXIS 3250 (NJ Super. Ct. Ch. Div. 2009). Both of these cases came before *Obergefell v Hodges* (135 S. Ct. 2584, 2600-01 (2015), which extended marriage to same sex couples in the United States . But as NeJaime persuasively argues, "the privileging of different-sex over same-sex couples and men over women in the legal regulation of the family" is still ubiquitous (2260).

[37] Ria Tabacco Mar, "Opinion: My Kid Has 2 Moms. Why Did She Say She's Thankful for 'Mommy and Daddy'?," *New York Times*, November 21, 2018, https://www.nytimes.com/2018/11/21/opinion/children-thanksgiving-gratitude-gay.html.

is different. That reinforces the notion that having a mother and a father is the norm"[38] and also that parents are "normally" genetically related to their children.

Those are not the same thing. Indeed, Tabacco Mar's story highlights the extent to which bionormativity is a mash-up of *heteronormativity* (families consist of mothers and fathers) and *biogenetic normativity* (families consists of parents who are genetically related to their children). The two are closely related.[39] Biogenetic normativity implies heteronormativity. But the opposite is not true: two families might equally buck biogenetic norms by having adopted children, while only one bucks the standards of heteronormativity (because one family is queer while the other is not). There are, then, plausibly two (closely related) social forces behind the interest in genetic knowledge, and it would be interesting to learn whether the interest is driven by biogenetic normativity or, more simply, heteronormativity (i.e. as a search for a "father" and less as the search for a *genetic* progenitor).[40] In many cases, the answer is surely "both," as illustrated by the following story:

> Emily and her mom found blue eyes, height, and musical abilities as traits that helped them make sense both of the donor and Emily herself. It did not matter that these traits might not really come from the donor. What mattered is that this ten-year-old had a place from which to understand that she too, like other children has a male progenitor whose significance is both tangible and positive.[41]

In light of all this, is it any wonder that people who do not fit the biogenetic mold are likely to develop an interest in acquiring genetic knowledge? If you are effectively told—through culture, law, institutions, people's comments, etc.—that you are missing something, you are very likely to want to find it. What Bartky says about the phenomenology of gender oppression plausibly applies in this context as well:

---

[38] Tabacco Mar, "Opinion."

[39] There is also what we might call the cultural demand for *racial homogeneity* between parents and children. As Russell puts it: "While the (heterosexual) family is seen as a site of gender difference, it is simultaneously expected . . . to be a site of racial sameness." Camisha A. Russell, *The Assisted Reproduction of Race* (Bloomington: Indiana University Press, 2018), 28. As Russell makes clear throughout her book, the expectation of racial sameness plays a big role in the choices that people make, and which are made available, in the context of donor conception.

[40] Thanks to Alice Maclachlan for discussions about the heteronormative component of bionormativity.

[41] Hertz and Nelson, *Random Families*, 38.

It is hard enough for me to determine what sort of person I am or ought to try to become without being shadowed by an alternate self, truncated and inferior self that I have, in some sense, been doomed to be all the time. For many, the prefabricated self triumphs over a more authentic self which, with work and encouragement, might sometime have emerged.[42]

Jean Benward, a psychotherapist who specializes in adoption and infertility, has seen this dynamic play out in her practice:

> The relatively narrow view of family currently in ascendance in North America is at the heart of one of the challenges the donor-conceived face in identity formation. A broader paradigm of extended kinship would allow donor-conceived individuals to create an identity that acknowledges different kinds of attachments—genetic and non-genetic.[43]

In the absence of that broader paradigm, your story is only complete, is only satisfying, if you know the answer to the question "Who are your genetic parents?" Other stories are deemed imperfect or lacking. Given that that's the game, it is not just understandable, but rational, to want genetic knowledge.[44] "The 'search for identity,'" says Katherine O'Donovan, "... does not exist in a vacuum."[45]

2.2. The bionormative prejudice

We are partway to making the case that donor-conceived people's interest in genetic knowledge is insidiously morally problematic. According to the

---

[42] Bartky, *Femininity and Domination*, 24. Bartky's use of the word "truncated" as a description of the "pre-fabricated" self that is foisted upon her as a woman is particularly resonant in light of Velleman's description of the lives of people who lack genetic knowledge as "truncated."

[43] J. Benward et al., "Identity Development in the Donor-Conceived Child," in *The Right to Know One's Origins: Assisted Human Reproduction and the Best Interests of Children*, ed. Juliet Ruth Guichon, Ian Mitchell, and Michelle Giroux (Brussels: ASP, 2012), 174.

[44] To the extent that donor-conceived people cannot conceive of "non-genetic" ways to engage in the task of identity formation, then they are plausibly subject to hermeneutical injustice. Miranda Fricker, *Epistemic Injustice: Power and the Ethics of Knowing* (New York: Oxford University Press, 2007), chapter 7. We will hear from someone who fits this description below (p. 147).

[45] Katherine O'Donovan, "'What Shall We Tell the Children?' Reflections on Children's Perspectives and the Reproduction Revolution," in *Birthrights: Law and Ethics at the Beginnings of Life*, ed. Robert Lee and Derek Morgan (New York: Routledge, 2003), 101–2. O'Donovan here is specifically talking about the "search for identity" in adoptees.

argument so far, the bionormative conception of the family reigns supreme in society at large and is also reflected in the attitudes of many parents of donor-conceived children. It is no surprise that donor-conceived children would come to internalize the idea that genetic relatedness *really* matters (for more than health reasons) and so develop an interest in it. In other words, it is highly plausible that many donor-conceived people's interest in genetic knowledge is a function of the bionormative conception of the family.

Even if that's right, it is not enough to show that the interest is insidiously morally problematic. For that we need the further claim that the bionormative conception is a form of prejudice. For those who think the biogenetic family is the gold standard or Platonic form of family forms, the bionormative conception of the family does not evince prejudice. It reflects the truth. In other words, if you think the bionormative conception of the family is more or less right, it won't strike you as problematic that the interest in genetic knowledge is a function of it. Instead, you'll think that donor-conceived people really *are* missing something important and that their family structures are derivative or second best.

But if you are not sympathetic to the bionormative conception of the family, then it will seem plausible that it is a form of prejudice. After all, a *superiority claim* is part of the bionormative conception of the family: "Families formed via biological reproduction . . . are, for that reason, superior to families formed in other ways." If that claim is unjustified, then the bionormative conception of the family evinces prejudice toward non-traditional families. It unjustifiably valorizes a particular family form. If that is right *and* donor-conceived people's interest in genetic knowledge is a function of the bionormative conception of the family, then the interest in genetic knowledge has the hallmarks of an insidiously morally problematic interest. It is both a function and a reflection of prejudice, and further entrenches it.

This brings the objection to the Significant Interest view fully into focus. The Significant Interest view depends on the ideas that (a) satisfying one's worthwhile significant interests makes one's life go better and (b) parents have a weighty reason to help their children satisfy their worthwhile significant interests. If insidiously morally problematic interests are not worthwhile and the interest in genetic knowledge is insidiously morally problematic, then the Significant Interest view is in trouble. This is the Bionormativity objection.

3. Three initial responses to the Bionormativity objection

3.1. First response: insidiously morally problematic interests are worthwhile

One response to the Bionormativity objection rejects the claim that morally problematic interests are not worthwhile *in the relevant sense*. That Significant Interest view was presented before we made the distinction between baldly immoral and insidiously morally problematic interests. With that distinction in hand, I might concede that the interest in genetic knowledge is (usually) insidiously morally problematic, but argue that the sense of "worthwhile" I've intended all along was meant to exclude only baldly immoral interests. Satisfying baldly immoral interests doesn't make one's life go better (and even if it did, it certainly doesn't follow that parents have a weighty reason to help their children satisfy those interests). Insidiously morally problematic interests are another matter altogether (according to this response). We might think that satisfying insidiously morally problematic interests does make one's life go better and that, as such, parents have a weighty reason to help their children satisfy even their insidiously morally problematic interests.

This response might appear *ad hoc*, but I don't think it is. It is an open question whether satisfying baldly immoral interests is good for the interest holder. But as we have seen, it often makes prudential sense to have and satisfy morally insidious interests. As a result, the general principle that enjoins parents to help promote their children's overall well-being applies to helping children satisfy insidiously morally problematic interests (as well as entirely morally unproblematic interests).

If that's right, then the Well-Being Principle applies as much to insidiously morally problematic interests as to entirely unproblematic interests. Moreover, precisely because satisfying insidiously morally problematic interests is not substantially harmful to others, while also being prudentially valuable for the interest holder, parents plausibly have a weighty reason to help their children satisfy interests of this kind.

But promoting these kinds of interests should be done *grudgingly* precisely because the interests are a response to oppressive circumstances. Even if we grudgingly concede that it is best for a child to satisfy an insidiously morally problematic interest, we should not just take her interest as given and then focus on how best to help her satisfy it. We should, as Haslanger puts it, "make every effort to disrupt the hegemony of the schema."[46] In other words, we should work to make the world such that the insidiously morally problematic interest is not on the menu (let alone one that it is reasonable to adopt given the menu).

This first response to the Bionormativity objection leaves the Significant Interest view in a relatively weak state. It works for the world as we find it, but it grants that we should work to have a world where the Significant Interest view has no purchase. Maybe that is precisely the right conclusion!

3.2. Second response: the importance of "having a say" in one's identity construction

Another argument we could make in response to the bionormative objection appeals to the argument in chapter 4. One central idea there was that having genetic knowledge can be a part of someone's task of determining their identity. An interest in genetic knowledge could be part of someone's understanding of themselves, of how they go about answering the question "Who am I?" (even if it is in no way required for answering that question).[47] So, even if the interest is insidiously morally problematic, it can still be an important part of a person's identity, of who they are.[48]

What does this matter? As Matthew Smith has argued, a person's cares—their significant interests, in my language—are "those traits through which a person *has a say* in who she is as an individual. By 'listening' to individualizing traits, we 'listen' to the individual, and do not supply for that individual our own picture of who she is."[49] Identity determination is a central human activity, a broad prudential good that can be specified in any number of ways. Healthy identity determination is, as we saw, both an epistemic activity (a matter of having an accurate conception of oneself) *and* an agential activity (a matter of choosing to construct one's identity one way rather than another). It is the latter element of identity determination that matters here. What a person cares about will largely dictate how the agential part of identity

---

[46] Haslanger, "Family, Ancestry, and Self," 181.

[47] I have couched the claim here as a psychological one. But the point in chapter 4 was also, indeed largely, normative: genetic knowledge can *properly* play a role in identity determination. It is a legitimate, even if optional, source of self-understanding. For now, this point doesn't matter, but it will in a bit.

[48] Non-metaphysically speaking.

[49] Matthew Noah Smith, "The Importance of What They Care About," *Philosophical Studies* 165, no. 2 (September 1, 2013): 301, https://doi.org/10.1007/s11098-012-9929-0.

determination unfolds. If we care about someone, then we have reason to support how they healthily determine their identities, including what they see as significant for answering the question "Who am I?" (within the constraints of the epistemic side of the task). And this is true even if one of the interests they build their identity around is insidiously morally problematic.

Is it, though? For we might wonder: Is identity determination around genetic knowledge *healthy* identity determination if the interest in genetic knowledge is a function of bionormative prejudice? If the person's interest in genetic knowledge is a result of their unjustifiably valorizing genetic knowledge—if, that is, they are genetic chauvinists—then why think that what we have here is an example of healthy identity determination? Indeed, the person's identity construction doesn't seem to meet the epistemic side of healthy identity determination, namely that it be largely accurate. The person we are imagining now thinks that genetic knowledge *really matters* in a way that it doesn't. Granted, that is not quite like believing you are Napoleon. But even so, the person is determining their identity around an interest that is grounded in a belief that just isn't accurate. What's healthy about that?

We might insist that even here, parents have some reason to support their child's identity determination. It is, after all, *who the child is*. It is not unreasonable to think that it is in the child's best interest to have their parents support them in their own self-conception, even if that self-conception is partly built around an insidiously morally problematic interest. But as with the first response to the bionormative objection, the response here is quite weak. And it is weak for the same reason. It is a grudging response to an imperfect world, to an interest that shouldn't arise in the first place, according to this way of seeing things. Given that it *does* arise, (maybe) parents have a reason to support their child in how she determines her identity. But, once again, they should do so with an eye to disrupting the problematic schema that made this particular form of identity determination so salient to their child in the first place.[50]

3.3. Third response: there really isn't that bionormative prejudice

The lesson from the first two responses is this: even if there is a case to be made that the Significant Interest view can accommodate insidiously morally

---

[50] And again: maybe this is the right conclusion.

problematic interests, that accommodation is highly conditional since it is made as a concession to a morally problematic schema. If we think the conclusion should be stronger—that intended parents ought to *non-grudgingly* help their child satisfy a foreseeable interest in genetic knowledge—then we need to consider another way of responding to the bionormative objection, one that shows that the interest in genetic knowledge is not insidiously morally problematic.[51] How might we show that? The third response to the insidious problem aims to show that even if the interest in genetic knowledge is a function of societal norms, attitudes, *etc.*, those norms do not evince bionormative prejudice.

So, is there widespread bionormative prejudice? As we have seen, genetic chauvinists will say "no," not because they deny the superiority claim but because they think it is true. But if we are not genetic chauvinists (and as I argued in chapter 4, we shouldn't be) then this route for responding to the bionormative objection isn't available. Instead, we can put pressure on the idea that common sentiments about the value of genetic ties amount to prejudice.

In order to do that, let's return to the claim that the bionormative conception of the family evinces an unjustified valorization of genetic ties. There is a stronger and a weaker version of that claim. The stronger version maintains that the way in which we value genetic relatedness has *no* rational basis, that it is not reflective of anything worthwhile outside of the problematic social structure that gives it a kind of distorted value. The bionormative conception of the family, in highly prizing genetic ties, valorizes something that is, in fact, evaluatively inert or close to it. On this view, "mere" facts of genetic relatedness are no more significant than facts about the number of blades of grass on my lawn.[52]

If the strong claim is right, then it seems very likely that people's interest in genetic knowledge is insidiously morally problematic. What could explain people's interest in genetic knowledge other than societal structures that valorize genetic relatedness in a way that is itself not rationally grounded (since there is no rational basis for valuing genetic relatedness)?

The argument in chapter 4 put paid to this line of thought since it showed that there is genuine value to determining one's identity along the "genetic

---

[51] The ideas in this section and the next are especially indebted to discussions with Emily Tilton, Andrée-Anne Cormier, Samantha Brennan, Olivia Schuman, Carolyn McLeod, and Alice MacLachlan.

[52] Bearing in mind, once again, that we have set aside the Medical Reasons view.

route," as I called it. There are, in other words, prejudice-independent rational grounds for valuing genetic ties. The genetic route is one way, among many, of healthy identity determination.

But there is a weaker, and in my view far more plausible version, of the bionormative prejudice claim: while there might be something valuable about genetic relatedness, society tends to *over*value it compared to other bases of family relatedness. This conception of the bionormative prejudice is perfectly consistent with the view that the genetic route, as I've called it, is valuable and it can be rational to pursue it apart from social norms that valorize genetic ties. The prejudice, according to this view, emerges in the idea that genetic relatedness is uniquely or especially valuable.

Suppose someone wanted to argue that bionormative prejudice in the weaker sense is not as widespread as it seems. How might they do it? They might start by making a distinction between the two following ideas: 1. *the dominant cultural attitude is to highly value genetic ties* and 2. *the dominant cultural attitude is to chauvinistically value genetic ties*. It is beyond doubt that the first claim is true. But that is not enough, by itself, to get to the second.

The person who wants to argue that bionormative prejudice is not widespread might use that inferential gap to make their case. To see how, let's return to some of the examples I discussed above. Some clearly evince genetic chauvinism. But one might argue that others don't, or at least, not obviously. Consider again the song "Hey Sister!" The whole song is basically a genetics-based answer to the question "Who am I like?" But it does not, on its own, suggest that there couldn't be other, equally valuable modes of establishing meaningful family relationships. Walter Martin could write another song, "Hey Other Sister!," that takes as its inspiration the unique goods that come with adoption. The two songs could happily exist side by side. More generally, at least some of the myriad cultural expressions of the value of genetic ties do not, on their own, imply that other modes of constituting families or determining one's identity are worse. They are simply not modes that most people engage with in any real way.

But the idea that genetic ties really matter is surely often implied in a weaker sense. The abundance of cultural products that valorize genetic family ties and the comparative absence of cultural products that valorize other kinds of family ties are no doubt partly explained by the fact that people have a kind of default assumption that genetic ties *really* matter and that other kinds of family ties are a mere approximation.

But even here, it is easy to overplay the (admittedly strong) hand. To see why, consider a personal example. Anyone who lives in North America—with just a few exceptions—is inundated with Christmas *everything* for about one month every year: songs, advertisements, religious messages, *etc.* It is impossible to escape. It is utterly dominant. It is clearly an event of massive cultural importance to most people, one which most people highly value. Not me: I'm Jewish[53] As a kid, I felt really left out. The days around Christmas were some of the worst of the year—I couldn't call any of my friends to play and none of them ever called me. We never had a tree.

No doubt many people who celebrate Christmas are Christmas chauvinists. Indeed, the annual conservative media frenzy about the so-called War on Christmas is both a symptom and a cause of a subculture in America that explicitly conceives of the United States as a Christian nation and, in ways both subtle and not so subtle, denigrates non-Christian traditions. But many people are not Christmas chauvinists. There are many people who simply do Christmas without ever giving any real thought to the value of other traditions. Perhaps they should. But that does not make them Christmas chauvinists. They do not overvalue Christmas with respect to other traditions. Indeed, if asked to think about other traditions, many would happily accept that they are equally worthwhile (it's just not what *they* do). And then there are others who are aware of other traditions and think them equally valuable to their own. They will say, "This is how *we* do things. But Hanukkah is equally wonderful! There's no part of me that thinks it is somehow of lesser value. It's just not what we do." Indeed, I take it that this was precisely the attitude of basically all my friends.[54]

Someone might claim something similar is going on when it comes to how lots of people think about the value of genetic ties. For many people, a significant portion of identity determination is built around genetic ties. It is *their* default mode of answering the question "Who am I?" No doubt many people *are* chauvinistic about it. It is not just that they cannot imagine their own lives without genetic knowledge. They also think that those who don't have it are, *ipso facto*, worse off. But many people don't have this attitude at all, either because they simply haven't given any thought to questions about the value of non-genetic modes of identity determination, or they *have* and don't believe that the genetic path is more valuable than other paths of identity

---

[53] Well, at least not me as a kid. I'm married to a cultural Protestant and have two kids, so I now celebrate Christmas every year. I love it. Sorry Mom and Dad.

[54] Although not the boy in Cubs Scouts who told me that people who celebrate Hanukkah are stupid.

determination. So, perhaps we should not treat it as utterly obvious that genetic chauvinism is as widespread as it seems.

In response to this line of thought, someone might claim that the fact that the dominant cultural attitude highly values genetic ties is enough to make that culture oppressive for people who lack genetic knowledge.[55] That, in turn, would make the interest in genetic knowledge insidiously morally problematic (assuming it is a function of the oppression).

Whether this response succeeds will depend on what we mean by calling a culture "oppressive." The concept has no single, precise meaning, so there isn't much point in trying to sharply delineate its contours. But it is worth noting that our bionormative culture does not have some of the hallmarks of Frye's conception of an oppressive culture. It is not clear, for example, that donor-conceived people are systematically confronted by double binds as a result of being donor-conceived, or that there are structures in place that "tend [. . .] to the immobilization and reduction"[56] of donor-conceived people as a group, or that bionormativity "is a product of the intention, planning and action for the benefit" of the dominant group in order to "secure privileges that are available" to members of that group.[57] At the very least, whatever the real hardships donor-conceived people face by living in our bionormative culture, they are not comparable in severity to the kinds of hardships women and people of color face (to focus on the two groups that informed the discussion at the start of this chapter).

Even so, we should reject this response to the bionormative objection for two reasons. First, even if bionormative prejudice in the form of people's attitudes is not as common as some might think, the presence of prejudice is not just a matter of people's hearts and minds. It is also a function of being subject to prejudicial structures, i.e. structures that effectively prejudge what counts as normal or how things ought to proceed. As we saw above, there

[55] Would this weaker sense of oppression still count as "cultural imperialism"? It's not clear to me that it would. A key feature of cultural imperialism, as Young conceives it, is that when the dominant group encounters other groups, "[t]he dominant group reinforces its position by bringing other groups under the measure of its dominant norms" and that "[g]iven the normality of its own cultural expressions and identity, the dominant group constructs the differences which some groups exhibit as lack and negation." Young, *Justice and the Politics of Difference*, 55. Suppose that in response to encountering non-dominant groups, the dominant paradigm is willing to shift, to acknowledge difference in a way that doesn't conceive of the non-dominant other as (normatively) lacking something. Then, while the dominant group will remain dominant (and so continue to shape the culture at large), the "mere" dominance seems to lack a key and especially problematic feature of cultural imperialism. I think we should be hesitant to conceive of cultural imperialism in a way that *any* social norms, institutions, practices that reflect a dominant cultural practice are thereby oppressive.

[56] Frye, *The Politics of Reality*, 10–11.

[57] Frye, *The Politics of Reality*, 12.

are bionormatively prejudicial structures (our examples were from medicine, education, and the law) which create friction for people whose families do not fit the bionormative mold. In the absence of prejudicial attitudes on the part of people involved, these structures may not be *degrading* to people whose families do not fit the bionormative mold. But the structures are nonetheless dominant in a way that makes people whose families do not fit the bionormative mold have to explain themselves when they fill out a form, or deal with a legal matter, or complete a school assignment.

Perhaps there is room to argue that if people's interest in genetic knowledge is a function of dominant but non-degrading social structures, then the interest is not insidiously morally problematic. According to this way of thinking, the dominant, non-degrading bionormative structures generate a relatively innocent form of path dependence. They shine a light, so to speak, on the genetic route of identity determination, but not because of any commitment to the superiority of that path. It is no surprise, in light of where the light shines, that people become interested in the genetic route. But that doesn't render the interest morally problematic.

Maybe we should be wary of interests that are a function of even innocent path dependence.[58] But the more forceful response to the above line of thought is to deny that the interest in genetic knowledge is just a function of innocent path dependence. And this takes us to the second reason for rejecting the idea that bionormativity does not evince prejudice: even if many people don't harbor bionormative prejudice in their hearts and minds, it is still ubiquitous. For in order for a prejudicial attitude to be ubiquitous, it just needs to be the case that it will show up basically anywhere. And in order for that to be case, there just needs to be some people who harbor the attitude.

The idea is not that donor-conceived people are confronted with genetic chauvinism at every turn, in every domain of their life, at every moment. The idea rather is that they are wildly unlikely to go for any meaningful length of time without encountering it in some guise, even if it is in the relatively mild form of having to confront "the shocked responses of people who—on learning that I don't know my donor—could not understand how I could be comfortable with this and believed I must be harboring hurt about

---

[58] Such an argument might appeal to Mill's defense of the value of individuality and the dangers of conformity in *On Liberty*. John Stuart Mill, *"On Liberty" and Other Writings*, Cambridge Texts in the History of Political Thought (Cambridge: Cambridge University Press, 1989), chapter 3.

it."[59] So, we should reject the claim that bionormative prejudice in the form of denigrating attitudes isn't that common. It *is* common in the sense that matters: people who are subject to it will encounter it often throughout their lives.

The upshot is that we live in a world that is rife with structures and people that evince and reinforce the dominance of the bionormative picture of the family. In light of that, responding to the bionormative objection by claiming that people's interest in genetic knowledge is not a function of bionormative prejudice because there isn't much bionormative prejudice is not a promising strategy.

3.4. The fourth (and best) response to the bionormative objection

Recall that we are looking for a response to the Bionormativity objection which shows that donor-conceived people's interest in genetic knowledge is not (usually) insidiously morally problematic. We have rejected a strategy that grants that bionormativity is present widely present in society, but denies that it is oppressive or prejudicial.

That leaves us with a fourth response, which maintains that the interest donor-conceived people tend to have in genetic knowledge is not a function of bionormative prejudice *in the sense that would make it insidiously morally problematic*. What we need is an account of what it means to say that the interest (indeed any interest) is a *function* of oppressive norms.

It is no doubt true that if we lived in a society where *nobody* cared about genetic relatedness, then donor-conceived people probably wouldn't care either. But that is not enough to show that people's interest in genetic relatedness in our world is a function of bionormative prejudice in any interesting sense. Almost all of our interests—indeed, all of them if we consider the specific form they take at a particular place and time—are a function of the society we live in. If society were radically different, our interests (considered in all their particularity) would be as well.

So what would make the claim—that an interest in genetic knowledge is a function of bionormative prejudice—interesting? To answer that question,

---

[59] Anonymous Us, "I Have Never Met My Donor 'Father' and I Have No Desire to Do So," October 31, 2011, https://anonymousus.org/i-have-never-met-my-donor-father-and-i-have-no-desire-to-do-so/.

let's return to the kinds of gendered interests I talked about at the start of the chapter. I gave the example of a 15-year-old girl wanting a nose job. It will be helpful to have some other examples on the table as well. Consider the interest that some women have to be "thin" or that other women have to undergo breast-augmentation surgery because they believe it will make them more attractive. These interests clearly bear the marks of insidiously morally problematic interests I identified above: they reflect the problematic attitudes that gave rise to the interest and are themselves an expression of those problematic attitudes. Moreover they are not unreasonable given the oppressive circumstances women finds themselves in. This was a key mark of insidiously morally problematic interests.

The question is whether an interest in genetic knowledge is, structurally speaking, the same as the above examples.[60] On the face of it, it is. But now consider the following question: Do the interests we're looking at remain rationally intelligible in *non*-oppressive circumstances? When we consider the particular gendered interests on the table, the answer is "no." The oppressive schema, and only the oppressive schema, renders those interests intelligible. This is what makes having the interests unqualifiedly a shame. It would be better if the world were such that the interests had no home, so to speak.[61] The goal is to change the schema so that the interests no longer have any rational ground. The claim is not that we couldn't imagine *some* non-oppressive possible world where wanting a nose job or breast augmentation was rationally intelligible. It is easy to do if we're willing to go to Sci Fi La La Land, a favorite stop of philosophers everywhere.[62] We might imagine a world where, for whatever reason, getting a nose job or breast augmentation had nothing to do with oppressive beauty standards and everything to do with unlocking the secrets of the universe. But such a world is nothing like ours. The point is that, in a world like ours, the gendered interests we're considering are not rationally intelligible absent the oppressive schema they are currently a part of.

The interest in genetic knowledge is not like this. As I argued in the previous chapter, there is genuine value to determining one's identity along the "genetic route." If that's right, then the interest in genetic knowledge is rationally intelligible quite apart from the bionormative social milieu

---

[60] Special thanks to Emily Tilton for helping me think through these ideas.

[61] As Benson puts it, "What feminine socialization aims to instruct women about the value of their appearance is *untrue*." In other words, the interests in conforming to most societal standards of beauty have no ground outside of those standards. Benson, "Autonomy and Oppressive Socialization," 388, emphasis added.

[62] I don't mean to knock it. I like it there too sometimes.

that surrounds it. Crucially, it is not rationally intelligible only in Sci Fi La La Land, but in our world and for creatures like us (indeed, especially for creatures like us given facts about how we come to exist and end up as we are). The interest in genetic knowledge is not a function of bionormativity in the sense that it is *only* the oppressive schema that makes the interest rationally intelligible. Someone, however, might wonder why *this* is the relevant sense of what makes an interest a function of oppression. Surely what matters is that, as a matter of fact, a person's interest in genetic knowledge is a response to bionormative prejudice and not that, in principle, it *could be* rationally grounded apart from it.

I have two answers to this line of thought. First, what *leads* to an interest is often different from what *now rationally grounds* it. A particularly inspiring music teacher might lead to someone's lifelong passion for jazz. But what grounds that passion now, what makes it the case that they continue to have a passion for jazz, are features of the music itself. Likewise, even if bionormative prejudice gives rise to some people's interest in genetic knowledge, it could be that what now grounds the interest floats free of the prejudice and instead reflects the (optional prudential) value of genetic knowledge itself.

This is not just armchair speculation. Consider two very different accounts from donor-conceived people about why they want genetic knowledge. Here is Bill Cordray's first-person account of his life as a donor-conceived person:

> Why do I want to know my identity, my family genealogy, my heritage? Ever since I began speaking in public about my donor conception, I have been asked this question countless times. *And each time, I'm astounded.* My right to know my genetic father is so crucial to my sense of identity that I'm shocked that anyone should ask such a question. Why wouldn't I want to know? *Wouldn't anyone else want to know?*
>
> In fact, I'm outraged that I'm in this position. How can a physician withhold from me my history? No legislature or court gave a gynaecologist *the power to deny me my basic identity.*[63]

Cordray's interest in genetic knowledge clearly expresses genetic chauvinism. The genetic route is not just his preferred route of identity determination but,

---

[63] In Juliet Ruth Guichon, Ian Mitchell, and Michelle Giroux, eds., *The Right to Know One's Origins: Assisted Human Reproduction and the Best Interests of Children* (Brussels: ASP, 2012), 40, emphasis added.

in effect, the only route. It is essential to his "basic identity," because it is basic for anyone's identity. It is something that anyone else would want to know.[64] It seems safe to say that Cordray's interest in genetic knowledge is grounded in bionormativity.

Consider, by way of contrast, Olivia Pratten's account of her long, and ultimately unsuccessful, legal battle in Canada to learn the identity of her donor. In a section entitled "Why I Would Like to Know My Biological Father" Pratten says:

> We each choose to construct our identities in different ways. Some people embrace identity through their families and through their biological ties. For some, identity is constructed solely from a cultural group affiliation or from other non-blood relationships. For many more, it's a combination of both.[65]

Pratten here beautifully articulates a commitment to genetic pluralism. And in stark contrast to Cordray's account, Pratten's description of identity determination emphasizes what I have called its agential aspect: "We each *choose to construct* our identities in different ways." In Pratten, we find a donor-conceived person who rejects genetic chauvinism, but still has a significant interest in acquiring genetic knowledge.

If Pratten's attitude is common, many donor-conceived people's *current* interest in acquiring genetic knowledge is not grounded in internalized bionormativity, even if bionormativity is rampant and even if it gave rise to the interest.[66] Is Pratten's attitude common? It is difficult to say. There are some hints that it is. Consider something we saw back in chapter 3: the little social science that has been done on donor-conceived children suggests that "curiosity" is the most common answer for why people want genetic knowledge. That is not the answer one would expect if people thought they were missing something utterly fundamental for identity determination. On the

---

[64] It is, perhaps, not surprising that Cordray thinks of identity determination primarily in epistemic terms—"Why do I want to *know* my identity. . . ?"—as though his true identity is out there, just waiting to be discovered.

[65] In Guichon, Mitchell, and Giroux, *The Right to Know One's Origins*, 50–51. Pratten goes on to to offer an autonomy-based account of why she wants to know who her donor is: "I aim to gain control of how I choose to construct my identity."

[66] Moreover, views like Cordray's often seem to come with some of the confounding factors I discussed in chapter 2. Indeed, Cordray's story about how he became interested in acquiring genetic knowledge begins like this: "This story was based on a lie. For 37 years, I did not even know that I was conceived through donor insemination."

other hand, the tendency of people to tell simplistic—or outright false—stories about the genetic origins of various traits (like a Jewish sense of humor) suggests that people often see genetic knowledge as a font of self-knowledge that it just cannot be.

But the empirical question (of whether Pratten's attitude is common) brings me to my second response to the idea that the interest in genetic knowledge is insidiously morally problematic if it in fact arises from bionormativity. Whether Pratten's attitude is common or not misses the larger point. The interest in genetic knowledge can—in our world—be rationally grounded apart from the oppressive schema it is embedded in. As a result, we should not discount the interest or aim to get rid of it. Rather, we should aim to change the schema so that the interest can more easily, and more often, manifest in an unproblematic way. The interest in genetic knowledge might routinely grow in unhealthy soil. But unlike genuinely insidiously morally problematic interests, it does essentially depend on it. This really matters. For in the case of both genuinely insidiously morally problematic interests and the interest in genetic knowledge, we should aim to change the soil. But the goal of doing so is different in the two cases. When it comes to genuinely insidiously morally problematic interests, we aim to change the soil so we can stop the interest from growing altogether. But when it comes to the interest in genetic knowledge, we should change the soil so that the interest can properly flourish as a potential, albeit optional, source for self-knowledge.

How we might go about changing the bionormative soil is a massive and massively important question. I take a small step toward answering it in chapter 8. The goal in this chapter has been to show that the interest in genetic knowledge is *not* insidiously morally problematic in a way that causes problems for the Significant Interest view. I have argued that people's interest in genetic knowledge *is* worthwhile in the relevant sense. It is an interest that can manifest in a healthy way and which parents should take seriously (in a non-grudging manner). They should neither discount it, nor aim to quash it. If that's right, then the Significant Interest view is safe.

6

Tipping the Scale

> There are always reasons. You can get reasons in any chor bazaar, any
> thieves market, reasons by the bunch, ten chips a dozen.
>
> —Salman Rushdie, *The Moor's Last Sigh*, 2011

Suppose you buy the arguments of the previous three chapters: you believe
that donor-conceived people are likely to develop a worthwhile significant
interest in acquiring genetic knowledge and that, as a result, intended parents
have a weighty reason to use an open donor.

You might still think, "Nu! So what?"[1] Why? Because, to borrow a phrase
from David Sobel, "reasons are cheap."[2] I have reasons to do all kinds of things
that, all things considered, I shouldn't do. I have a reason to stop writing this
book and binge-watch *Gilmore Girls* (again), but all things considered I have
more reason to plug away on the book. Maybe something similar is true for
intended parents who plan to conceive with donated gametes. Maybe they
have a weighty reason to use an open donor. But what we really want to know
is whether they have a decisive reason to use an open donor. And to know
that, we need to know what reasons there might be to use an anonymous
donor. Might intended parents have reasons to use an anonymous donor
that—singly or together—outweigh the reason to use an open donor?

It is not hard to think of philosopher-style examples where someone has
a decisive reason to use an anonymous donor. Perhaps the fate of the world
depends on it! But what we really want to know is whether, *in general*, there
are reasons to use an anonymous donor that outweigh the reason to use an
open donor. I will argue that, in general, there are not. To be clear: I think

---

[1] Did you know you can speak Yiddish?

[2] David Sobel, review of *Slaves of the Passions*, by Mark Schroeder, Notre Dame Philosophical
Reviews, April 25, 2009, https://ndpr.nd.edu/news/slaves-of-the-passions/. Sobel uses the phrase
as a shorthand for a view developed and defended by Mark Schroeder, *Slaves of the Passions*
(New York: Oxford University Press, 2007).

Conceiving People. Daniel Groll, Oxford University Press. © Oxford University Press 2021.
DOI: 10.1093/oso/9780190063054.003.0006

there *are* good reasons many intended parents might have to use an anonymous donor. I just don't think those reasons generally outweigh the reason to use an open donor. Or so I will attempt to show.

Before we get going, it's important to remember that back in chapter 2 we established that parents generally should not keep *the secret*. That is, parents should disclose to their donor-conceived child that they are donor-conceived, even if the donor is anonymous. So the question now is not whether intended parents have decisive reason to use an open donor versus *using an anonymous donor and never disclosing*. Rather, the question is whether the weighty reason identified by the Significant Interest view provides a decisive reason to use an open donor given that, in general, parents should disclose to their child that he is donor-conceived.

1. Intrinsic versus extrinsic reasons

In answering this question, we need to distinguish between at least three classes of intended parents:

1. Those who live in places where anonymous donation is prohibited. These parents still have the option of conceiving with anonymous gametes by either going to a country that allows for anonymous donation or ordering anonymous sperm for home insemination.[3]
2. Those who live in places, like the United States, where anonymous and open donation are both allowed.
3. Those who live in places—like France—where anonymous donation is required.

The burden of using an open donor differs for the three classes of intended parents.

Someone in France, for example, might find using an open donor especially burdensome. This burden would probably not justify using an anonymous donor if the resulting person would be denied a profound prudential good. But the Significant Interest view doesn't make that claim. Instead, it claims that the resulting child stands to have a significant subjective interest frustrated. Now this is not nothing! But even so, lots of people have some of

---

[3] See, for example, https://dk.cryosinternational.com/how-to/how-to-order-donor-sperm.

their significant subjective interests frustrated. It is not the end of the world. So perhaps in France there are reasons to use an anonymous donor that countervails the reason to use an open donor identified by the Significant Interest view.

It is important to see, though, that this potentially countervailing consideration is extrinsic to the practice of donor conception. Extrinsic considerations are generated by features of particular legal or regulatory frameworks for donor conception. These features might highly constrain the choices available to intended parents who live under particular frameworks. The potentially countervailing reason to use an anonymous donor, which exists in France, would be removed altogether by changing France's regulatory framework. The same is true for many other burdens related to cost or access that intended parents anywhere might encounter.

Extrinsic countervailing reasons can be contrasted with intrinsic countervailing reasons. These are reasons that parents might have against using an open donor that are *not* the result of a particular regulatory or institutional framework for donor conception.[4] They are reasons we can expect to find in any (realistic) donor-conception regime.

The distinction between extrinsic and intrinsic countervailing considerations leads to the following question: In thinking about whether the Significant Interest view has identified a decisive reason to use an open donor, should we consider both extrinsic and intrinsic potential countervailing reasons or only the latter? My goal is to show that there are not, generally speaking, intrinsic countervailing reasons. Limiting the focus in this way will not get us to the conclusion that intended parents, no matter where they find themselves, generally have decisive reason to use an open donor. But it will get us to the conclusion that there is nothing about the practice of donor conception itself that (usually) generates a countervailing reason. This is a significant result since it provides at least some reason to think that regulatory frameworks that generate extrinsic (potential) countervailing reasons should change, thereby making the choice to use an open donor widely available and relatively frictionless.[5]

---

[4] I consider examples of potential intrinsic countervailing reasons in the next section.
[5] I consider what the regulatory implications of my view are in chapter 8.

2. In search of intrinsic countervailing reasons

What potential intrinsic reasons (henceforth, just "reasons") could there plausibly be for not using an open donor? We already looked at one obvious candidate back in chapter 3. If there were good reasons to think that having genetic knowledge would be bad overall for donor-conceived people, then the Significant Interest view would be easily defeated. That's because it appeals to the likely prudential benefits of having genetic knowledge. If it turns out those benefits are swamped by the harms that come from gaining genetic knowledge, then the rationale I've identified to use an open donor has little force indeed. As we saw in chapter 3, however, the evidence suggests that, in general, it is not bad for donor-conceived people to gain genetic knowledge. We can, then, put this possible countervailing intrinsic reason aside.

What others could there be? The Significant Interest view itself suggests one. Intended parents *themselves* might have a significant subjective interest in their child not acquiring genetic knowledge. Not all intended parents will have this interest. But, as we know from the discussion of why people keep *the secret*, some certainly do. So now we might wonder: If a donor-conceived person's significant interest in acquiring genetic knowledge generates a weighty reason to use an open donor, does an intended parent's significant interest to the contrary generate a reason to use an anonymous donor?

The answer depends in part on why the parent has an interest in using an anonymous donor. If it's because they believe having genetic knowledge will, overall, be bad for their donor-conceived child, then, for reasons we've just seen, the interest is not well-grounded. But an intended parent's interest in using an anonymous donor might not be child-centered at all. Rather, they might be worried about the impact on *them* of their child acquiring genetic knowledge.

We can separate this issue into two separate concerns. First, intended parents might be concerned about the *emotional* impact on them if their child is in a good position to acquire genetic knowledge. To put it simply, they might worry that it will seriously compromise their own happiness. Second, intended parents might be concerned that planning for a child's foreseeable, future interest in genetic knowledge runs counter to their (the parents') *values*. Separating out the source of the concern in this way is somewhat artificial, since acting contrary to one's values is likely to cause emotional distress. Moreover, inasmuch as people value their own emotional well-being, acting in a way that causes emotional distress to oneself will run counter to one's values to some extent. But we can still keep the rationales separate. It is the difference between someone who says, "My child acquiring genetic knowledge will be very emotionally difficult for me and *that* is why I have an interest in their not acquiring it," and "Quite apart from whatever emotional distress it will cause me, my child acquiring genetic knowledge runs counter to my values." Let's consider these possibilities in turn.

There is no doubt that having one's child track down her donor will often be emotionally difficult and complex for everyone. The child's social parents must contend with their child coming to know someone else who bears a kind of parental relationship[6] to the child, which the child herself sees as significant in some way.[7] The question is whether there is good reason to think that, in general, such emotional difficulties will be so great (for the parents) that it justifies using an anonymous donor. While there is no doubt that the emotional distress is real for some parents of donor-conceived children, there is also some evidence that it is usually short lived:

> According to Pamela, Celeste, as the nongenetic mother, has had moments of distress about all the focus on inherited traits that accompanied seeing Justin and Michael [the donor] together for the first time: "She said, 'God, all this gene stuff, I don't know how I fit into this.'" However, Pamela also suggested that "the next day, it was sort of like gone." [. . .] Several genetic parents . . . reported on how distressed their same-sex partners had been at the moment of meeting the donor or donor siblings. Each of them also commented that the distress was short-lived and that, on the surface at least, everything went back to normal.[8]

---

[6] It is in the very least a *genetic* parental relationship. Whether it is something more is an issue I take up in chapter 7.

[7] As Freeman et al. observe, the question of "language and the problem of how to describe each other and [the] relationships" looms large for donor-conceived children, their families, and the donor when it comes to linking donor-conceived children and donors. Tabitha Freeman, John B. Appleby, and Vasanti Jadva, "Identifiable Donors and Siblings," in *Reproductive Donation*, ed. Martin Richards, Guido Pennings, and John Appleby (Cambridge: Cambridge University Press, 2012), 288. In their research on donor-conceived children and families, Hertz and Nelson report:

> Some parents—and this was often the nongenetic parent—feared that contact with genetic strangers would highlight the issue of genes in a household that is predicated on the assumption that nurture is as important as—if not more important than—nature. Other parents worried that their child might be more interested in connections.

See Rosanna Hertz and Margaret K. Nelson, *Random Families: Genetic Strangers, Sperm Donor Siblings, and the Creation of New Kin* (New York: Oxford University Press, 2018), 52.

[8] Hertz and Nelson, *Random Families*, 91.

One thing to note is that how much of an impact acquiring genetic knowledge has for the relevant parties (parents, the donor-conceived person, and the donor) depends in part on how they *see* the significance of the acquisition. If the parent of a donor-conceived person thinks that his relationship with his child will be torn asunder if the child acquires genetic knowledge, then it is very plausible that it *is* more likely to be torn asunder. In other words, someone's concerns about the negative effects of their child having genetic knowledge can be self-fulfilling. Another important point is that some parents of donor-conceived children are actively interested in giving their kids access to genetic knowledge.[9] This is not to say they are entirely unconflicted or that it's always an easy process. The point is that it is not inevitable that parents of donor-conceived children will experience strong, negative emotions should their child acquire genetic knowledge.

What all this suggests is that how someone responds to the prospect of their child acquiring genetic knowledge is at least partly a matter of how they *choose* to relate to it. In other words, figuring out whether you are likely to have a strong, negative emotional reaction to your child acquiring genetic knowledge is not just a matter of *predicting* your future behavior, as though you are a passive bystander to your own attitudes on the matter. It is at least partly a matter of how you choose to orient yourself to the prospect of your child acquiring genetic knowledge. As a result, whatever worries an intended parent has about the negative emotional impact for them of using an open donor should not be taken as a given, i.e. as a factor that is outside their control and which needs to be priced into the costs of using an open donor. Rather, the presence of such concerns gives intended parents a reason to change their views about the significance (to them) of their child acquiring genetic knowledge so as to minimize the likelihood of a negative outcome for themselves and their child. I don't mean to suggest that people can simply decide to approach the situation in a way that minimizes the possibility for a negative emotional outcome. People are limited in their ability to directly control their emotions. But we do have some control. We can work to look at things differently, to get used to an idea, to prepare ourselves for something coming down the pipe so that it won't affect us as negatively as it otherwise might.

Even so, it is not unreasonable for intended parents to wonder whether they will suffer as a result of their child acquiring genetic knowledge. This

---

[9] See, for example, Freeman, Appleby, and Jadva, "Identifiable Donors and Siblings," 280.

is all the more true if that knowledge leads to contact, and possibly an on-going relationship, with the donor. The latter is not something that even those parents who help their child gain genetic knowledge tend to want.[10] So, concern about the negative emotional impact on the parents is an intrinsic (parent-centered) reason against using an open donor.[11] Just how weighty it is, though, is another matter we'll turn to presently.

Let's turn to the second way a parent might have a significant interest in not helping her child gain genetic knowledge, namely that providing such help runs counter to the parent's *values*. Someone who is committed to the idea that the interest in genetic knowledge is insidiously morally problematic—because it evinces and entrenches a kind of bionormative prejudice about what families ideally should be like—will have a values-based, significant interest in not helping their child acquire genetic knowledge. Sympathetic though they may be, they will nonetheless see their child's interest as morally problematic, as a symptom of a society that denigrates families like theirs. Helping their child acquire genetic knowledge, by using an open donor, for example, will make them complicit with a schema they oppose.

This line of thought returns us to the arguments of chapters 4 and 5, which aimed to show that donor-conceived people's interest in acquiring genetic knowledge is not generally insidiously morally problematic. If that is right, then it is questionable whether the parent's values-based significant interest in using an anonymous donor has much, if any, weight at all, let alone enough to countervail the reason to use an open donor that I've argued for.[12] The parents' values are misguided. There are difficult questions here about whether, and how much, weight to give to people's misguided consciences.

---

[10] Tabitha Freeman et al., "Gamete Donation: Parents' Experiences of Searching for Their Child's Donor Siblings and Donor," *Human Reproduction* 24, no. 3 (2009): 509.

[11] Just a reminder that "intrinsic" here doesn't mean that it is always present with donor concep-tion, but that it is a consideration that is *not* a function of a particular regulatory or institutional framework of donor conception. So, the fact that many intended parents might not worry about the negative emotional impact on them doesn't mean that the worry isn't "intrinsic" in my sense.

[12] Notice that if it's not, then we don't need to appeal to the fact that the *parents* have a values-based significant interest in using an anonymous donor in order to block the conclusion that they should use an open donor. Why? Because the Significant Interest view itself depends on the claim that in general donor-conceived people's interest in acquiring genetic knowledge is worthwhile (i.e. at least non-trivial and not morally problematic). If the child's interest really is insidiously morally problem-atic, then *there is no reason to countervail* in the first place. In other words, if the parent's value-based significant interest has force in virtue of being right about the moral insidiousness of the interest in genetic knowledge, then we don't need to appeal to the parent's significant interest to block the con-clusion that parents should use an open donor. We never would have got to that conclusion in the first place. So pointing to a parent's (purportedly) *justified*, value-based significant interest in not helping his child acquire genetic knowledge just returns us to the question of whether a donor-conceived person's interest in genetic knowledge is generally morally problematic.

Diving into them would take us too far afield. Instead, we can say the following: if a donor-conceived person's interest in acquiring genetic knowledge is not, in general, insidiously morally problematic, then that person's parents shouldn't see it as morally problematic. If they do, then they should change their minds. If they don't, then we are dealing with a less than ideal situation generated by the *parents'* morally problematic position, i.e. that they shouldn't help their child as a matter of misguided conscience—though of course they don't see their conscience as misguided![13]

Suppose, however, that we imagine the parent's values differently: he does not think that, in general, the interest in genetic knowledge is morally insidious. He acknowledges that the interest is worthwhile in at least the minimal sense of being non-trivial and not morally problematic. But *he* does not value such ties. Nor does he want to structure part of his life, or his family's life, around an interest in those ties. Indeed, we can suppose that he has a significant interest in promoting a conception of family ties that does not depend on genetic ties. This, we might say, is a project of his. His child's foreseeable, likely significant interest in acquiring genetic knowledge runs counter to this project.

Surely this version of the parent's significant interest generates a reason not to use an open donor. Though he does not see his child's interest in acquiring genetic knowledge as worthless, it nonetheless runs counter to the parent's values. He has chosen to plant his flag, so to speak, in territory that does not focus on genetic connectedness. He understands that his child can justifiably pursue an interest in acquiring genetic knowledge. But the parent has a significant interest in not helping. And this generates a reason not to use an open donor.

3. The weigh-in: assessing the contenders

We now have two candidates for intrinsic reasons against using an open donor. The first is that putting one's child in a position to get genetic knowledge will open some parents up to a negative emotional experience. The

[13] But even if the parents' misguided significant interest carries some weight, it is hard to believe that it would outweigh the reason to use an open donor generated by a child's *legitimate* interest in acquiring genetic knowledge. And even if it did, appealing to the importance of letting parents follow their misguided consciences provides a weak argument for why people sometimes don't have a decisive reason to use an open donor. It is weak because it must acknowledge that *ideally* the parents would have *no* such reason for the simple reason that, ideally, their values would not be misguided.

second is that putting one's child in a position to acquire genetic knowledge involves acting against one's values. Are there others? No doubt. But I think they will all have the same general shape. Some parents will have a strong (subjective) interest in their child not having genetic knowledge, and—assuming that the interest is not totally misguided—this will generate *some* reason not to use an open donor.

The question is whether a reason of this kind is enough to outweigh the reason to use an open donor. I don't think it is. In order for it to really provide a decisive reason to use an anonymous donor it is not enough that, from the impartial point of view, it is as weighty as or even just a little bit weightier than the reason to use an open donor. Instead, it must be considerably weightier.

Why? The explanation has nothing to do with the specific reasons in play, but rather the following principle: when parents' and children's legitimate interests conflict, the parents' interests ought to be discounted *because they are the parents' interests*.[14] Let me put it another way. Suppose parents find that their legitimate interests conflict with their child's legitimate interests. The principle says this: the fact that the parents' interest is the parents', and the child's interest is the child's, means that the parents' interest counts for less than it otherwise would. This idea is captured in the very common thought that parents should (always) act in their children's best interests. Now that is a very strong version of the norm I'm interested in. It implies that parents should apply a discount rate of 100% to their own interests when any of their children's interests are at stake. I am not advocating for that view, which I think is (obviously) mistaken.[15] Nonetheless, parents' have *some* obligation to prioritize their children's interests over their own. If the legitimate competing interests are even roughly equal considered apart from whose interest is whose, then when we assign the interests to the relevant parties—the parents and the children—the parents' interest counts for considerably less than the child's.

As I have said, the disparity in the competing interests' weight is a function of a general truth about how to weigh the interests of parents and their children. But that disparity is plausibly amplified by four features of the specific interests in play here. First, intended parents can—or at least should—see in

---

[14] Just how much it should be discounted—and how precisely we might determine the discount rate (let alone figure out a way to quantify the non-discounted weight of the relevant interests in play)—is not something I attempt to answer.

[15] I discuss it in some detail in chapter 8. See Daniel Groll, "Four Models of Family Interests," *Pediatrics* 134, Supplement 2 (2014): S81–S86; John Hardwig, "What about the Family?," *Hastings Center Report* 20, no. 2 (1990): 5–10.

advance that their child is likely to develop an interest in acquiring genetic knowledge. They cannot, therefore, treat the occurrence of the child's interest as an unanticipated disruption of their competing interest in the same way they justly might react to some other, utterly unpredictable significant interest their child might develop ("I've decided to join the circus!"). Intended parents of a donor-conceived child cannot reasonably claim that working to satisfy the child's interest imposes a surprising cost on them.

Second, intended parents—but not the child—voluntarily step into the situation where there might be a conflict between their significant interests and the child's. This is true in some sense for every situation where parents' interests conflict with their kids'. Anyone who decides to become a parent is choosing to put themselves in a situation where, at least sometimes, their interests will conflict with the child's. The same is not true of the child, who did not choose to be in the child-parent relationship. Perhaps this asymmetry explains the general principle that parents' interests should be discounted in the face of competing interests of their child. But even if that's so, the *particular* interests at play here make the asymmetry even more pronounced. Here's why: people who choose to have children know, in a general way, that there will be times when their interests conflict with their child's. But often it is hard to know in any specific way when the conflicts will arise and what they will be about. Such is not the case with the interests we're focused on here. People who plan to create a child with donated gametes *and* have a significant interest in their child not acquiring genetic knowledge can—at least they should—foresee a probable future conflict between their interests and the child's. They are, in effect, voluntarily taking on the mantle of this particular conflict.

The third point is closely related to the second. We just noted that parents voluntarily step into the (likelihood of) conflict, while the child does not. But that way of putting it doesn't make clear that the *parents themselves* are centrally responsible for foisting this conflict on the child. Again, there's a sense in which all parents are responsible for foisting onto their child whatever conflicts of interests occur between them (since they brought the child into existence). But that's not the point I'm interested in here. The point I want to make is that there's a way in which parents of donor-conceived children bear a direct responsibility for the conflict we're talking about. To see what I mean, consider, once again, our fan of dB drag-racing. Let's call her Dora. It is true that Dora's parents' decision to have and raise a child is part of the story of how Dora came to be interested in dB drag-racing. But it is a distal part of the story. An account of Dora's interest that stopped at the fact she was conceived would be no account at all! We need to hear far more to understand why she is interested in dB drag-racing, and whatever we hear may well have nothing to do with her parents. The same is probably not true when it comes to explaining a donor-conceived person's interest in acquiring genetic knowledge. If we ask, "How did you become interested in acquiring genetic knowledge?" we will learn a lot—although not everything—when the person says, "I am donor-conceived." The decision to conceive with donated gametes plays a large role in making it foreseeable that the donor-conceived person will likely develop an interest in genetic knowledge. So, when parents of donor-conceived people intentionally conceive a child with donated gametes, *they* play a large role in generating the likely future interest in genetic knowledge that makes up one side of the conflict between the child's interest and the parents'.

Finally, unlike with many other significant interests a child might have, the parents of a donor-conceived child have a tremendous amount of control over whether this interest will be satisfied. Their decision to use an open donor is probably the central factor in whether their child will fulfill a future interest in acquiring genetic knowledge.

So, intended parents who have a significant interest in their child not acquiring genetic knowledge (1) should foresee that their child will likely develop an interest in genetic knowledge, (2) have voluntarily put themselves in a position of (likely) conflict with the child, (3) are directly responsible for the child being in the (likely) conflict, and (4) have a huge amount of control over whose interest will be satisfied (theirs or the child's). These four features of the conflict taken together, if not singly, plausibly require parents to discount the weight of their own interest even more than is required by the general obligation of parents to discount their interests in the face of their child's conflicting interests. Whatever discounting of parental interests is generally required will be amplified when parents can foresee the likelihood of conflicting interests *and* have voluntarily stepped into the conflict *and* have introduced the other party into the conflict *and* are basically in control of which side's interest will prevail.

Here's what this all means. Intended parents might well have a significant, legitimate interest in using an anonymous donor. It might even be true that the interest is more or less proportionate in strength to their child's interest in obtaining genetic knowledge. But unless that interest is a *lot* weightier than the child's interest in having genetic knowledge, it will not outweigh the reason to use an open donor articulated by the Significant Interest view. And insofar as no other candidate countervailing reasons exist, then the weighty reason to use an open donor identified by the Significant Interest view provides a *decisive* reason. In other words, intended parents should, all things considered, use an open donor because their child is likely to have a significant, worthwhile interest in acquiring genetic knowledge.

7

The Donor's Responsibilities

> My four year old, when asked by a friend at day care why she has two
> mums and no dad, told her that her dad was eaten by a shark.
>
> @BakeKater, 2020

I have argued that intended parents normally have decisive reason to use an
open donor. But where is the donor in all this? Must he choose to be an open
donor? In fact, some readers might have even more fundamental questions
about donors' responsibilities: Do donors incur *parental* responsibilities to
the child? And, if they do, does that imply that being a donor is morally impermissible in the first place?

My main goal in this chapter is to show that gamete donors are not parentally responsible, even if it's true that gamete donation is the kind of thing
that "triggers" parental responsibility. My second goal is to show that even if
donors are not parentally responsible, they should choose to be open donors.

1. Gamete donors and parental responsibility: having my cake and eating it too

Are gamete donors parentally responsible for their genetic offspring? You
might think that's the same as asking whether gamete donors are *parents* to
their genetic offspring. But that way of putting things invites confusion because of the different ways people use the word "parent."

To illustrate this point, consider the following exchange I witnessed between a gamete donor and his friend:[1]

---

[1] Truly. I'm not making it up.

Conceiving People. Daniel Groll, Oxford University Press. © Oxford University Press 2021.
DOI: 10.1093/oso/9780190063054.003.0007

DONOR: So, I'm donating gametes to Jennifer [a mutual friend].

CLOSE FRIEND: You'll be the child's father!

DONOR: No, I definitely won't be its father.

CLOSE FRIEND: If there's one thing you definitely *will* be, it's the kid's father.

It might seem like the donor and his friend were disagreeing, but it's more likely they were invoking different notions of what it means to be a parent or, in this case, a father. There's at least one sense in which the donor is undeniably the child's parent: he is the child's genetic parent. This is what the friend likely meant when he said "If there's one thing you definitely will be, it's the kid's father!" But when the donor denied he will be the child's parent, he was probably invoking a different notion of parenthood. To see why, consider what's going on when a child says something like "How could you do that to me? My own father!" The child here is pointing to the fact that there is a sense of "parent" that consists of having moral obligations of a particular kind. What it *is* to be a parent, in this sense, is to stand in a particular kind of normative relationship to the child. To be a parent, normatively speaking, is to be *parentally responsible* for the child. Asking whether a gamete donor is a parent is ambiguous, whereas asking whether he is parentally responsible is not.

Some philosophers claim the gamete donors do not incur parental responsibilities toward their genetic offspring.[2] They argue for this conclusion by giving a general account of how someone incurs parental responsibilities and then show that it doesn't implicate gamete donors as normative parents in the first place. Joseph Millum, for example, argues that parental responsibilities are "artificial duties," inasmuch as their "acquisition depends upon the existence of social conventions regarding their acquisition."[3] To put Millum's view too simply, parental responsibilities are incurred by engaging in acts that, through social convention, constitute incurring parental responsibilities. For Millum, gamete donation is *not* such an act:

---

[2] Tim Bayne, "Gamete Donation and Parental Responsibility," *Journal of Applied Philosophy* 20, no. 1 (2003): 77–87; Joseph Millum, "How Do We Acquire Parental Responsibilities?," *Social Theory and Practice* 34, no. 1 (2008): 71; Jason Hanna, "Causal Parenthood and the Ethics of Gamete Donation," *Bioethics* 33, no. 2 (2019): 267–73. Hanna does not in fact accept the causal theory of parenthood that he discusses in the article. Rather, he attempts to show that proponents of the causal theory can defend themselves from the "too many parents" objection to the view (and that such a defense implies that gamete donors do not incur parental responsibilities).

[3] Millum, "How Do We Acquire Parental Responsibilities?," 75.

Gamete donors do not acquire parental responsibilities because their acts, though they may eventually lead to children, are not considered to constitute taking on responsibilities. (If gamete donors reasonably believe that they are not going to be held parentally responsible, then they have not taken on parental responsibilities by donating.)[4]

On this view, donors (typically) never incur parental responsibilities. I'll call this the Never Responsible camp.

On the other side are those who argue that donors *do* incur parental responsibilities. This conclusion, unsurprisingly, is argued for by offering a general account of how someone incurs parental responsibility and then showing that it *does* implicate gamete donors.[5] But there is a crucial split among people who claim gamete donors incur parental responsibility. Some think that parental responsibilities can be fairly easily passed on to the intended parents.[6] Others think they cannot.[7]

This difference is grounded in a disagreement about the nature of parental responsibility. If you think parental responsibility demands that someone must lovingly raise the child himself or herself,[8] then it becomes clear why parental responsibility cannot be easily transferred. If *you* are on the hook for lovingly raising a child, it's not clear how you could pass that obligation to someone else. Gamete donors, according to this view, are forever parentally responsible for their genetic offspring. I call this the Forever Responsible camp.

But you might think that, at least initially, parental responsibility consists of something considerably more minimal, namely the responsibility to ensure that *someone* lovingly raises the child.[9] If that's right, then the person

---

[4] Millum, "How Do We Acquire Parental Responsibilities?," 81.

[5] I give an example of one such theory, which I provisionally accept, below.

[6] Elizabeth Brake, "Willing Parents: A Voluntarist Account of Parental Role Obligations," in *Procreation and Parenthood: The Ethics of Bearing and Rearing Children*, ed. David Archard and David Benatar (New York: Oxford University Press, 2010), 151–177; David Archard, "The Obligations and Responsibilities of Parenthood," in *Procreation and Parenthood: The Ethics of Bearing and Rearing Children*, ed. David Archard and David Benatar (Oxford University Press, 2010), 103–127; Giuliana Fuscaldo, "Genetic Ties: Are They Morally Binding?," *Bioethics* 20, no. 2 (2006): 64–76. Elizabeth Brake or David Archard. Fuscaldo, Giuliana. "Genetic ties: are they morally binding?." *Bioethics* 20, no. 2 (2006): 64–76. Although Bayne is in the *Never Responsible* camp, he argues that even *if* donors incurred parental responsibilities, they could be easily transferred.

[7] David Benatar, "The unbearable lightness of bringing into being." *Journal of Applied Philosophy* 16, no. 2 (1999): 173–180. Rivka Weinberg, *The Risk of a Lifetime: How, When, and Why Procreation May Be Permissible* (New York: Oxford University Press, 2016), 71.

[8] Weinberg, *The Risk of a Lifetime*, 49.

[9] Archard, "The Obligations and Responsibilities of Parenthood," 104. I'm using the terminology of "parental responsibility" differently than Archard does. He calls the responsibility to ensure the

who starts with parental responsibility can pass on the considerably more demanding responsibility of lovingly raising the child to someone else. Gamete donors, according to this view, might initially be parentally responsible, but they pass on the more demanding duty to lovingly raise the child to the intended parents. I call this the Initially Responsible camp.

My first goal in this chapter is to carve out space for a new camp, which I'll call the Prospectively Responsible camp. The key thought is this: when it comes to gamete donation, there is a gap between the action that triggers parental responsibility and those responsibilities actually coming "online." The presence of this gap opens up the possibility—and, I will suggest, actuality in almost all cases—that gamete donors are never actually parentally responsible. There is (usually) never a time when the donor's genetic child exists and the donor is parentally responsible for it. In this way my view is different from the Initially Responsible and Forever Responsible camps, which both accept that gamete donors incur parental responsibilities, while disagreeing on the nature of those responsibilities.[10]

Why isn't my view just part of the Never Responsible camp? There are two reasons. First, as I noted above, advocates of the Never Responsible camp think that gamete donation isn't the right kind of action to trigger parental responsibilities. I disagree. I accept that the right general account of how parental responsibility is incurred implies that donating gametes triggers parental responsibilities. Second, I think gamete donors incur a certain set of responsibilities by donating—prospective parental responsibilities—but that donors can transfer these responsibilities before they mature into actual parental responsibilities.[11] So, on my view, donors incur a kind of proto-parental responsibility by donating. There is something about gamete

child is lovingly raised by someone the "parental obligation" and the responsibility to lovingly raise the child the "parental responsibility."

[10] It could be that some people in the Initially Responsible camp would want to put themselves in the Prospectively Responsible camp once I've spelled out the implications of "the gap." That's fine. As far as I know, the presence and relevance of "the gap" have not been discussed in the literature on parental responsibility.
    [11] The position I develop here is similar to that developed by Bayne, who argues that sperm donors have "potential parental responsibilities" that are transferred when they donate their gametes. Bayne, "Gamete Donation and Parental Responsibility," 83. See also Fuscaldo, "Genetic Ties." Fuscaldo says that with gamete donation a "pre-conceptual transfer of parental duties is understood" between donor and prospective parents (74), but it is not clear to me whether she thinks the *understanding* that parental duties *will be* transferred is pre-conceptual or that the duties themselves are pre-conceptually transferred (even though there is, as yet, nothing to be parentally responsible to!). If she means the latter, then I think she will agree with the position I argue for. But her discussion (73) of how her view differs from Bayne's makes me think she means the former.

donation that gets the ball rolling toward parental responsibility. This is something the Never Responsible camp denies.

So much for the conceptual differences between the camps. What are the practical implications of being in one camp rather than another? If the Forever Responsible camp is right, then gamete donors are, in effect, deadbeat parents and the whole practice should probably stop. The question of whether intended parents should use an open or anonymous donor quickly recedes to the background. The same is not true with any of the other three camps, since none implies that gamete donors are failing in their parental duties. What is at stake, practically speaking, between them?

Being in the Initially Responsible camp has a practical implication that neither the Prospectively Responsible nor Never Responsible have: the possibility of the donor refusing to pass on his parental responsibilities to the intended parents when the child is born.[12] According to the Never Responsible camp, the donor has no parental responsibilities to (refuse to) pass on. And according to the Prospectively Responsible camp (for reasons we'll get to), donors transfer their prospective parental duties well before there is a child on the scene to be responsible *to*. In other words, by the time the child is on the scene, the matter has been settled.[13]

But then what hangs on whether one is in the Never Responsible camp or the Prospectively Responsible camp? Practically speaking, I'm not sure. But this is, in a way, a *strength* of being in the Prospectively Responsible camp. This is because, as a member of this camp I can have my cake and eat it too. That is, I can accept that gamete donation is the kind of activity that triggers parental responsibilities (have my cake), but also avoid the conclusion that

---

[12] Or at whatever point we think the child comes to exist. I talk about this important qualification below (pp. 170–71).

[13] Once again, perhaps people I've placed into the Initially Responsible camp would place themselves into the Prospectively Responsible camp after reading my account of how it differs from the Initially Responsible camp. The key point I'm after is that prior discussions of transferring parental responsibilities have not noted the important distinction between being parentally responsible to an existing child and being *prospectively* parentally responsible to a child that *will* exist. The distinction is important in part because it allows us to bypass altogether the question of whether parental responsibility is the kind of thing that, when actualized, can be transferred. I say more about this below (p. 172). Separately, whether one thinks gamete donors are initially parentally responsible or only prospectively parentally responsible, there is no doubt that some procreators who end up transferring parental responsibility are initially parentally responsible. People who give their children up for adoption shortly after birth, for example, are initially parentally responsible. They might *plan* to transfer parental responsibilities to someone else, but they cannot in fact transfer the responsibilities before the child is on the scene (as evidenced by the fact that people planning to give their children up for adoption shortly after birth can change their mind).

gamete donors are ever parentally responsible (eat it too). But why should I want to have my cake in the first place?

There are two reasons. First, I am largely convinced by the theory of how people incur parental responsibility that I present in the next section and so not convinced by views—such as Millum's—according to which gamete donors stand outside the chain of parental responsibility altogether. Second, and more importantly, I want my cake for dialectical reasons. Here's what I mean: those who think gamete donors never incur parental responsibilities of any kind can simply skip ahead since, in their view, there's no question to deal with here about the transfer of parental responsibilities, prospective or actual. From their point of view, what I do in this chapter is, at worst, a waste of ink. But for those who think gamete donation does trigger parental responsibilities of some kind, failing to address whether and how transfer of those responsibilities is possible would constitute a massive gap in my argument. It is the latter group of people I want to address. I want to show that even if we accept a view about parental responsibility that is hostile to the view that gamete donors do not incur parental responsibilities, we can nonetheless conclude that they do not.[14] So, I'm going to present a theory that explains why donating gametes triggers parental responsibilities. But I will not argue for the theory or try to show that it is superior to accounts of how someone gets parental responsibility that don't implicate gamete donors at all. Instead, I will show that even if we accept this theory (have my cake), we can avoid the conclusion that gamete donors are parentally responsible (eat it too).

2. Incurring parental responsibilities

Rivka Weinberg's Hazmat Theory of parental responsibility offers a compelling and intuitive account of how parental responsibilities are incurred. According to Weinberg:

> Parental responsibility is incurred when we choose to engage in activities that put our gametes at risk of joining with others and growing into persons, and persons results from those activities. That is the Hazmat Theory of parental responsibility.[15]

---

[14] Thanks to Jason Hanna for helping me think about how to frame this point.
[15] Weinberg, *The Risk of a Lifetime*, 162.

As the name implies, Weinberg's theory is an instance of a more general theory of how (at least some) responsibilities are incurred: if you are in possession of, and have a high degree of control over, something that is hazardous, *you* are on the hook for what happens as a result of the hazardous thing, whether it be uranium, a pet lion, or gametes.[16] And to be sure, gametes *are* a hazardous material. In the right (or perhaps the wrong) circumstances they give rise to extremely needy beings with significant moral status.[17]

Hazardous materials impose a standard of care on the people that possess them. Just how high that standard is depends on the relative weight of the competing interests at play in situations where someone is doing something risky with the materials. As Weinberg notes—and as we all know too well these days—breathing is a risky activity. We might exhale materials that can make others sick. But our interest in breathing freely is, in general, considerably weightier than other people's interest in avoiding the common, but not serious, illnesses that our breathing might propagate. So, the "risky" activity of breathing generates a very low standard of care. Things are different, on the other hand, if we have a highly communicable, serious airborne disease. If it is serious enough, our interest in breathing freely, indeed in being free, might be outweighed by others' interest in not contracting the disease to the point where the state is justified in quarantining us.

When it comes to creating children, lots of what we do comes with the risk of our gametes "joining with others and growing into a person."[18] So, what risks are we permitted to take without being in danger of incurring parental responsibilities? Are we off the hook if we use a reliable method of birth control, but it fails? If we think that a vasectomy has worked when in fact it hasn't? If we have drunken sex without thinking about birth control at all? Fortunately, I don't need to wade into these waters. The crucial point for my purposes is that any plausible answer to these questions will put *intentionally using your gametes to create a child* on the "You're parentally responsible!" side of the line. And this is precisely what gamete donors do. They knowingly engage in an activity with their gametes for the purpose of creating a child.

---

[16] Weinberg, *The Risk of a Lifetime*, 60–61.

[17] The fact that the result of joining gametes is a being with significant moral status suggests that there is something inapt in thinking of gametes as hazardous materials. We typically think of hazardous materials as something with no potential upside, something to be avoided or not used at almost all costs. By that standard, gametes are not hazardous since they have a very significant upside: children! What is beyond doubt is that there are significant costs and burdens that come with children (precisely because they are so precious. If they were not, we could just ignore them). Thanks to Jennifer Lockhart for pushing me on this point.

[18] Weinberg, *The Risk of a Lifetime*, 60.

There is not only no attempt to avoid creating a child, but also an active effort *to* create a child. If anything counts as a gamete-involving activity that causes the gamete possessor to incur parental responsibility, gamete donation will. The whole point is to create a child!

3. Triggering parenthood

If we accept the Hazmat Theory of procreative responsibility,[19] then gamete donation is exactly the kind of thing that will lead someone to incur parental responsibilities. As we saw above, this has serious implications for the practice of gamete donation if you think parental responsibility is the kind of thing that cannot be transferred, not even initially. You'll be in the Forever Responsible camp along with Weinberg. If, however, you think parental responsibility, at least initially, is the kind of thing that can be transferred, then you'll be in the Initially Responsible camp.

Now, I've just signed onto a theory according to which gamete donation is the kind of thing that leads to parental responsibility. But I also think that gamete donors never actually incur parental responsibilities to their genetic offspring. How does that work?[20] To answer that question, consider another: *When* precisely do people become parentally responsible? Whatever the answer, it cannot be that people become parentally responsible before there is something to be parentally responsible *to*. This is not to say that you cannot incur responsibilities generated by the prospect that there *will be* someone for whom people will be parentally responsible. You can. But these earlier responsibilities are neither *parental* responsibilities nor are they owed to the currently non-existent child.

Why not? After all, people routinely talk about our duties to future generations. We often say that it is our duty to save the environment for the sake of future people. We might even say we owe it to them, though, of course, they don't as yet exist. So, why can't people be responsible—parentally or

---

[19] Weinberg's argument is more sophisticated than this inasmuch as she argues that (a) competing accounts of how parental responsibility is incurred are not plausible and (b) there is no way to get gamete donors off the hook without, at the same time, getting other kinds of procreators off the hook that, intuitively, are on the hook. Again, my goal is not to argue for the Hazmat Theory, but rather to show that even if we accept it, we can avoid the conclusion that gamete donors incur parental responsibilities. There are critics of the Hazmat Theory. I've already mentioned Hanna's critique. Another is Andrew Botterell, "Why Gametes Are Not Like Enriched Uranium," *Bioethics* 30, no. 9 (2016): 741–50.

[20] I am indebted to Jason Hanna for helping me think through the arguments of this section.

otherwise—*now* to future children they will have? There's no denying that we talk about our duties to future generations. But such talk obscures an important difference between our duties to existing people and our duties to future people. Suppose you have a duty to an existing person. And suppose that you can't transfer it. There is just one way you can avoid failing with respect to your duty: you must discharge it. But there are *two* ways you can avoid failing with respect to your duty to a future person: you can discharge the duty *or* prevent the person from coming into existence. We don't let future generations down by degrading the environment if we also decide to stop reproducing. But we do let a young person down if we degrade the environment.[21]

What this suggests is that, regardless of how we talk, all duties to future people are duties *in prospect*. They only come online when the people exist. It is often true that in order to ensure that we don't fail right away with respect to those future duties we need to do stuff before they come online. So duties in prospect (to future generations, for example) generate real duties now (to, for example, stop burning fossil fuels). But they are not strictly duties *to* the future people. They are, rather, something like duties to prepare for the duties to others we will, but do not as yet, actually have because the "others" don't exist yet. They are not owed *to* the future people since we could dispense with the future duties by not bringing them into existence.

So, there can be no parental responsibility prior to there being something that someone can be parentally responsible to. The next question is: *When* is there something to whom someone can be parentally responsible? That's not a question I will try to answer, except to note that it can't be before conception.[22] Prior to conception, there is nothing someone could plausibly be *parentally* responsible to. So, even if gamete donation is the kind of action that will lead a donor to incur parental responsibilities, the donor does not, indeed cannot, incur them at the time of donation. This is not meant to be a substantive moral claim, but rather a borderline trivial argument. You cannot be parentally responsible without there being something to be parentally responsible *to*.[23] There is nothing to be parentally responsible to at the

---

[21] And certainly we let them down if we kill them so that we get out of the duty to not degrade the environment.

[22] I don't mean to suggest that one becomes parentally responsible at conception. The point is just that that is the earliest possible time when one could become parentally responsible. Before that, there is nothing to be parentally responsible *to*.

[23] What about my gametes? The idea that I am responsible *to* (and not simply *for*) my gametes is already a stretch. The idea that I am *parentally* responsible to my gametes—that I am the parent of my gametes—stretches the notion of parental responsibility past the breaking point.

time of gamete donation. So gamete donors are not parentally responsible to anything at the time of donation. There is a gap between the time of donation and the time a donor *would* become parentally responsible. At the time of donation, donors are merely *prospectively parentally responsible*.

We can now see how gamete donation "triggers" parental responsibilities. Donating gametes is a little like lighting a fuse. It is (part of) the start of a process that is intended to end in the BOOM of a child. Somewhere along the way—perhaps only when the child is born, perhaps sometime before that—parental responsibilities will kick in. But they don't kick in when the fuse is lit.

Does this mean that prior to the point where the donor would become parentally responsible, he incurs no new or distinctive responsibilities? No. To see why, consider the following story:

> **Melvin's Dangerous Work:** Melvin is involved in a line of work that, for whatever reason, seriously degrades the health of his sperm: any child that results from them is very likely to live a short, painful life. The good news for Melvin is that he has no intention of creating children with his sperm. So the state of his sperm is, rightly, of no special concern to him. One day, however, Melvin decides he wants to have a child and resolves to get to work on creating one.

Surely it is not permissible for Melvin to keep working at his job. Given that he intends to start using his sperm to create a child, he is now responsible for the health of his sperm in a way that he wasn't before. Crucially, that doesn't mean that he needs to *preserve* his spermatozoa (although he'll certainly want to preserve some of them if he plans to conceive). He is not responsible *to* the spermatozoa themselves! Rather, he is responsible for the health of the sperm that will be used to create a child. So if he knows that some sperm will not be used to create a child—perhaps because he plans to masturbate—then he has no reason to care for it at all. But he needs to worry about the health of the sperm that could end up creating a child. He would do something very wrong indeed if, having decided to create a child, he continued his sperm-damaging work.

Like Melvin, donors have decided to use their gametes to create children. And like Melvin, having so decided, they incur responsibilities of care with respect to their gametes. The contours of those responsibilities are something I'll return to presently. The point now is just that at least by the time they donate—but probably from when they resolve to donate in the near term—donors incur responsibilities that are generated by the interests of the child they intend to create. But these are not parental responsibilities. Rather, they are *procreative* responsibilities.[24]

So here's where we are. Gamete donation is the kind of activity that triggers parental responsibility. But those responsibilities only come online when there is something someone can be parentally responsible to. Whenever it is, it can't be before the child is conceived. Until then, donors are only prospectively parentally responsible. That is to say, they will incur parental responsibility for the resulting child unless something happens to prevent it, e.g. the sperm clinic burns down.[25] Even so, prospective parental responsibility comes with procreative responsibilities, things that the donor must do *now* as a procreator (like ensuring that his gametes are not seriously degraded).

It is worth emphasizing that mere possession of gametes is not sufficient to make someone incur prospective parental responsibility or procreative responsibilities. The example of Melvin illustrates that nicely. So long as he is not in the business of creating children, he is neither prospectively parentally responsible to any future children nor need he be concerned about the health of his sperm.[26] I've already mentioned one condition that is sufficient for making someone prospectively parentally responsible and procreatively responsible: intending to use one's gametes in the near term for the creation of a child. There are no doubt other conditions, but they need not concern us since gamete donation flips at least one of the switches for prospective parental responsibility.

Notice that if this is right, then Weinberg's claim that gamete donors are perennially parentally responsible for their progeny faces a problem *even if* you agree with Weinberg that parental responsibility cannot be transferred. Even if the person with parental responsibility must be the one to lovingly raise the child, the presence of "the gap" opens up the possibility that *who will be parentally responsibility in the first place* can be transferred before the child is conceived.

---

[24] The distinction between procreative and parental responsibilities is made by Bayne, "Gamete Donation and Parental Responsibility," 84.

[25] Or they transfer their prospective parental responsibility. More on that in just a moment.

[26] At least not from the point of view of concerns about the future child that could result from them.

4. Transferring prospective parenthood

Is it possible to transfer prospective parental responsibility? To be clear, this is a moral, not a legal, question. We're wondering whether, morally speaking, gamete donors can transfer their status as prospective parent to someone else. And what about procreative responsibilities? Can those be transferred?

If there is no way for a donor to *responsibly* transfer their prospective parental responsibilities and procreative responsibilities, then they cannot permissibly do so. If, for example, a gamete donor knowingly transfers care of their gametes to someone who will cause them to degrade in a way that will seriously adversely affect the health of the child, then the donor has, to borrow a term from Weinberg, *recklessly*—and so impermissibly—transferred their procreative responsibilities.[27] Likewise, if a donor transfers their prospective parental responsibilities to someone who will not be sufficiently attentive to the future child's well-being they have done so recklessly. These responsibilities cannot be transferred willy-nilly; it must be done *responsibly*. As we've seen, prospective parental responsibility and procreative responsibilities are not the same. But for ease of reading, I'm going to discuss the transfer of both sets of responsibilities together under the banner of transferring prospective parental responsibilities since the basic question is the same: Can they be responsibly transferred?

We need to distinguish, once again, between intrinsic and extrinsic considerations.[28] Extrinsic considerations—either for or against the possibility of responsible transfer—are a function of *contingent* features of particular gamete donation regimes. Intrinsic considerations, in contrast, are those that are present given any (realistic) regime for gamete donation. So, for example, someone might claim that the current regime of gamete donation in the United States does not allow for the responsible transfer of prospective parental responsibilities. This is an extrinsic consideration against the possibility of responsible transfer, in the United States at least. By contrast, someone might think that there is no feasible system of gamete donation where responsible transfer of prospective parental responsibilities is possible.

The distinction between intrinsic and extrinsic objections is important because the latter are remediable. If it turns out that particular gamete donation practices prevent responsible transfer of prospective parental

---

[27] Weinberg, *The Risk of a Lifetime*, 72.
[28] I made this distinction back in chapter 1 and then again in chapter 6.

responsibilities, then we have reason to change those particular practices. The same is not true of intrinsic objections: no feasible change in a system of gamete donation will overcome those objections. From a philosophical point of view, the intrinsic considerations are more basic because they point to problems with any realistic system of donor conception.[29] So, are there intrinsic reasons to think that donors cannot responsibly transfer their prospective parental responsibilities?

Here is one contender: gamete donors have no say in who chooses their gametes. How, then, can they responsibly transfer prospective parental responsibilities given that who uses their gametes is out of their control? Surely knowing *who* will be parentally responsible for the resulting child is a precondition of responsibly transferring prospective parental responsibility.[30]

One thing to note right away is that many gamete donors *do* know who will use their gametes. Some people donate gametes to close friends or family.[31] It is true, though, that most donation happens at clinics and involves parties who do not know each other. The donation is impersonal, whether it is open or anonymous. So the narrower worry is that impersonal gamete donation precludes responsible transfer of prospective parental responsibilities because donors do not know who will receive their gametes.

Notice that the worry now sounds like an extrinsic objection. For we might ask: Why couldn't donors know—and, indeed, have a say in—who wants to use their gametes? My claim is not that they should know or have a say. That's a complex question. My point, rather, is this: if the objection to the possibility of responsibly transferring prospective parenthood is that donors do not know who is receiving their gametes, then that situation is in principle remediable.

But let's set that aside and focus instead on the following question: Why does responsible transfer require the donor to know who he is transferring prospective, and eventually full-blown, parenthood to? So long as gamete

---

[29] This is not to say that extrinsic considerations aren't hugely important. They certainly are. But considering and responding to them is more a matter of getting the policy, rather than the philosophy, right.

[30] David Benatar, "The Unbearable Lightness of Bringing into Being," *Journal of Applied Philosophy* 16, no. 2 (1999): 176. Benatar says: "It seems that we should judge as morally defective those gamete donors . . . who are willing to donate sperm or ova without even knowing the identity, let alone the details, of those who will rear their genetic children. That transference of responsibility strikes me as being far too cavalier."

[31] Benatar concedes that in such cases, the transfer might be permissible. Benatar, "The Unbearable Lightness of Bringing into Being," 178–79.

donors entrust their gametes to a system that reliably picks out people who will be adequate parents, then it looks like the donor responsibly transfers prospective parental responsibility.[32]

Once again, we might wonder whether any existing gamete donation regimes instantiate such a system. Some gamete donation companies in the United States are not exactly paragons of responsibility.[33] It is reasonable to doubt whether they can be trusted to act as reliable intermediaries in the distribution of prospective parenthood. But these are surely extrinsic reasons to think prospective parenthood cannot be responsibly transferred (in the United States). Once again, the lesson is that the system should change to overcome these problems and *not* that there is something wrong with donor conception as such.

Here is another candidate for an intrinsic objection to the possibility of impersonal gamete donors responsibly transferring prospective parenthood: donors cannot be certain that the child who will be created with their gametes will be adequately parented either in prospect or in actuality. And, the thought goes, if they cannot be certain of that, then they cannot responsibly transfer their prospective parental responsibilities. Notice that this objection sets the standard for responsible transfer very high indeed, far higher than we set the standard for people that intend to create children in the "traditional" way and then raise them. There is a crucial difference between the cases. "Traditional" intended parents don't seek to *transfer* their parenthood (prospective or actual). So you might think we're just not talking about the same thing.

Yes and no. It is true that transfer of parenthood is not typically an issue for "traditional" parents. But it is *not* true that the issues that arise when thinking about transfer of prospective parental responsibilities aren't equally present when it comes to "traditional" parenthood. For even in the "traditional" case, we can still ask: "Will the people raising the child be good enough parents?" The fact that the people raising the child are "traditional" parents doesn't make the question irrelevant. Indeed, it is a question that prospective

---

[32] I make no claim here about what is involved in being an adequate parent, although I am partial to Liam Shield's "Dual Comparative View" of what makes parents "good enough." Liam Shields, "How Bad Can a Good Enough Parent Be?," *Canadian Journal of Philosophy* 46, no. 2 (2016): 163–82.

[33] For a good overview of the concerns, see Rene Almeling, "Opinion: The Unregulated Sperm Industry," *New York Times*, November 30, 2013, https://www.nytimes.com/2013/12/01/opinion/sunday/the-unregulated-sperm-industry.html. Note, though, that the problems she discusses here do not include the companies giving gametes to inadequate parents. Rather, the companies themselves are often inadequate stewards of the gametes. I say a little more about this below.

"traditional" parents should—but I suspect often don't—ask themselves. Of course, the question is about *them*. They are not looking to transfer prospective parenthood to anyone else. But that doesn't change the fact that they too must consider whether the people who will parent the child—in this case themselves—will be adequate parents.

We can put the point this way: the standard for responsibly *transferring* prospective parenthood shouldn't be any different than the standard for responsibly *becoming* a prospective parent, even if the intention in the latter case is to raise the resulting child. In both cases, we need to be concerned with whether the resulting child will be adequately parented. If we say that gamete donation is acceptable only if we are all but certain that things will end well (enough) for the child (otherwise, donors could not transfer their prospective parenthood), then we should say the same thing about when it is acceptable to "traditionally" acquire prospective parenthood. If the "can't be certain" standard is used as an argument against impersonal gamete donation, then we need to seriously consider whether it implies that all procreation is impermissible.

In response to this line of thought, some might claim "traditional" intended parents can often be sufficiently confident that their child will have adequate parents in way that gamete donors cannot. If this is true, then we would have grounds to treat *becoming* a "traditional" prospective parent differently than *transferring* prospective parenthood to intended parents. But this response overestimates the extent to which "traditional" parents can be sufficiently confident about whether they will be adequate parents and underestimates the extent to which gamete donors can be confident that the intended parents who conceive with their gametes will be adequate parents.

Consider the first point. There is, no doubt, something intuitive to the thought that "traditional" parents are better situated than a donor to know that the resulting child will be adequately parented. As we have seen, "traditional" intended parents at least know who will be parentally responsible for the child (them!). So they at least are in a position to directly assess the likelihood that they will be adequate. The same is not true of impersonal gamete donors, who must trust that the system does a good job identifying people who will be adequate parents. But we have already dealt with this. If the donation system could pick out adequate parents as reliably as the "traditional" way of picking out parents, then what does it matter if "traditional" intended parents, but not donors, can directly assess the adequacy of the future parents?

Perhaps the answer is this: it is true that "traditional" intended parents, just like gamete donors, ought to ask "Will the future child be adequately parented?" But when donors ask this question, it is entirely epistemic. Donors are, in effect, trying to predict or forecast the likelihood of an independent event. The same is not true, though, of "traditional" intended parents. They are not just trying to *predict* whether they will be good parents, as though their own wills are not partly determinative of the answer. They can partly answer the question from a practical point of view by *intending* or *committing* to be good parents.[34]

This is a real difference. But it's not a difference that makes a difference. First, even if "traditional" intended parents ask the question "Will the child's parents be adequate?" from a practical point of view—one where they are considering whether to *commit* to being good parents rather than predicting that they will be—a full answer to the question is not merely practical. There is a significant epistemic element to the question that cannot be settled by intending to be a good parent (if only it were so simple!). "Traditional" intended parents need to ask whether, knowing what they know about themselves and their circumstances, they can confidently *predict* they will be adequate parents (even assuming they intend to be). No amount of committing to be an adequate parent will render a confident "yes" to that question.[35]

The second reason it doesn't make a difference is this: all that really matters is whether the children that result from the procreative choices we are considering are adequately parented. Suppose there's no reason to think the answer is more likely to be "yes" when we're dealing with "traditional" parents versus non-traditional parents. Why, then, should it matter that "traditional" parents can answer the question "Will the resulting child be adequately parented?" from a practical point of view while gamete donors cannot?

This way of posing the question brings to the fore what I think is often behind the idea that gamete donors cannot be sufficiently sure—even in a

[34] J. L. Nelson, "Parental Obligations and the Ethics of Surrogacy: A Causal Perspective," *Public Affairs Quarterly* 5, no. 1 (January 1991): 60.Thank you to Jenn Lockhart and Micah Lott for a very fruitful discussion on these matters and the argument of the next few paragraphs.

[35] Bayne, "Gamete Donation and Parental Responsibility," 83. This point is all the more true if becoming a parent can be personally transformative, i.e. radically change the kind of person you are (and so what matters to you), in the way L. A. Paul argues it can be. See Laurie Ann Paul, "What You Can't Expect When You're Expecting," *Res Philosophica* 92, no. 2 (2015): 149–70; Laurie Ann Paul, *Transformative Experience* (Oxford: Oxford University Press, 2014). Bernard Prusak considers the line of thought I advance here, but declares it "specious" for the reason that "one can hold oneself accountable in ways that one cannot hold others." The second thought is undeniably true, but I don't see why it renders the point I'm making specious. Bernard G. Prusak, *Parental Obligations and Bioethics: The Duties of a Creator* (New York: Routledge, 2013), 21.

well-regulated system of gamete donation—that their genetic offspring will be adequately parented. The idea is that, barring evidence to the contrary, biological parents will be adequate. But people are skeptical that a process that transfers prospective parenthood to a non-genetic, intended parent could ever do enough to ensure the resulting child is adequately parented. Behind this difference in approach, I suggest, is a latent privileging of biological parenthood according to which, in general, biological parents make for the *best* parents.[36]

Here's the problem with that idea: the data don't bear it out. Available evidence suggests that "traditional" parents are no better at parenting than nontraditional parents, particularly when the latter have conceived children with donated gametes. Here is Susan Golombok summarizing the research on this issue:

> The European Study of Assisted Reproduction Families included a group of 111 families with 4- to 8-year-old children who had been conceived through donor insemination, and found the quality of parenting in these donor insemination families to be similar to that of IVF families and *superior to that of natural conception families*.[37]

> With respect to psychological adjustment, not a single study has shown that children raised by lesbian mothers [who conceived children with donated sperm] are more at risk for emotional or behavioral problems than are peers from heterosexual homes.[38]

> Findings from the few empirical studies conducted so far show that gay fathers [who adopted children] provide a supportive family environment for their children and that their children flourish. [. . .] Golombok, Mellish, Jennings, et al.[39] reported more positive parenting and child adjustment in adoptive gay father families.[40]

---

[36] It is true that in most cases of donor conception, the resulting child is raised by one biological parent. But the privileging that I'm positing here comes with the idea that, ideally, children are raised by both biological parents and so, in general, you're shortchanging a child by removing them from a biological parent.

[37] Susan Golombok, *Modern Families: Parents and Children in New Family Forms* (Cambridge: Cambridge University Press, 2015), 103.

[38] Golombok, *Modern Families*, 66.

[39] Susan Golombok et al., "Adoptive Gay Father Families: Parent-Child Relationships and Children's Psychological Adjustment," *Child Development* 85, no. 2 (2014): 456–68.

[40] Golombok notes: "Investigations of parenting and child development in gay father families created through surrogacy have only just begun." Golombok, *Modern Families*, 191. What about the so-called Cinderella Effect, according to which there are "higher incidences of different forms of child abuse and mistreatment by stepparents than by biological parents" *because* of the lack of biological connection between stepparents and stepchildren? "Cinderella Effect," Wikipedia, August 8, 2020,

Perhaps more research will tell us something else.[41] But for now, I see no reason to think that impersonal gamete donors are generally in a worse position than "traditional" parents to know whether a child that results from their gametes will be adequately parented. If "traditional" prospective parenthood is often responsibly incurred, then we have no reason to think that it cannot be responsibly transferred by impersonal gamete donors on the grounds of uncertainty about whether the intended parents will be adequate.

So here's where we are. Gamete donation triggers parental responsibilities of a kind, namely the responsibilities of prospective parenthood. These responsibilities can be transferred, morally speaking, to another person who will live up to the duties of prospective parenthood. There might be extrinsic reasons for thinking that such a transfer is not responsible—and so not morally permissible—within the current gamete donation regime. But there are no intrinsic reasons for thinking that gamete donors cannot responsibly transfer their prospective parenthood. There is nothing about gamete donation itself—either personal or impersonal—that prevents the responsible transfer of prospective parenthood.

But whom can gamete donors transfer prospective parental responsibilities to? And when? Asked so broadly, the answers are simple: (1) to anyone who is willing to take on the role of prospective parent (and will do a good job) and (2) at any time before parental responsibility kicks in. But the general question doesn't capture the dynamics of gamete donation. Donors, in general, do not want to be parentally responsibly. Intended parents who

https://en.wikipedia.org/w/index.php?title=Cinderella_effect&oldid=971884222. Even if the effect is real, there is reason to think neither that it is nearly as pronounced as its proponents think nor that it has to do with a lack of genetic connection rather than other, social factors. See Gavin Nobes, Georgia Panagiotaki, and Kenisha Russell Jonsson, "Child Homicides by Stepfathers: A Replication and Reassessment of the British Evidence," *Journal of Experimental Psychology: General* 148, no. 6 (June 2019): 1091–1102; David J. Buller, "Evolutionary Psychology: The Emperor's New Paradigm," *Trends in Cognitive Sciences* 9, no. 6 (June 1, 2005): 280–82. Finally, there's a significant gap between a finding about stepparents and any conclusion that can be drawn about the quality of other kinds of non-biological parent.

[41] I have offered Golombok's summaries of the findings that she discusses in detail in her book. She is also very clear about the limitations of the research that have produced these findings. See, for example, Golombok, *Modern Families*, chapter 2. Prusak cites what would seem to be conflicting evidence about how donor-conceived people fare from Elizabeth Marquardt, Norval D. Glenn, and Karen Clark, *My Daddy's Name Is Donor: A New Study of Young Adults Conceived through Sperm Donation* (New York: Institute for American Values, 2010). For some serious concerns about this study, see Wendy Kramer and Eric Blyth, " 'My Daddy's Name Is Donor': Read with Caution!," *BioNews*, July 9, 2010, https://www.bionews.org.uk/page_92455; John Corvino, "My Daddy's Name Is 'Donor,'" blog, June 4, 2010, https://www.johncorvino.com/2010/06/04/my-daddys-name-is-donor/.

use donated gametes do want to be parentally responsibly. So the question is this: Given that gamete donors are prospectively parentally responsible, how and when does the transfer of prospective parental responsibilities of parenthood end up with the intended parents?

Let's start with the case of known gamete donation. The "how" question is easily answered: the donor directly identifies the intended parent(s) as the people on the other end of the transfer of prospective parental responsibilities. If we stick with the Hazmat Theory of parental responsibility, then one of the intended parents is already prospectively parentally responsible in virtue of voluntarily contributing their gametes. And depending on how we choose to unpack the notion of a "hazardous material," the person who gestates the child—who could be different than either of the gamete providers—will also be a prospectively parentally responsible.[42] But we needn't worry about who among the intended parents starts out as prospectively parentally responsible. This is because even if the intended parents are already prospectively parentally responsible, there's no reason to think a donor cannot transfer *their* prospective parental responsibility to people who already have it. The situation is no different than three people who are jointly responsible for a piece of property. One member of the party can transfer their responsibility to the other two. Whereas before, three people rightly had a say about what happens to the property, only two do after the transfer. So, it is no objection to the schema I've developed to point out that intended parents (either one or both) already start as prospective parents. Donors can still transfer *their* prospective parental responsibilities to the intended parents.

The more difficult question, in my view, is "*When* can transfer of prospective parental responsibilities take place?" We already know that it cannot happen after parental responsibilities kick in since, at that point, the responsibilities are no long prospective.[43] I have avoided offering an account of when that happens, except to note that the earliest possible time that could be

---

[42] Interestingly, Weinberg does not count the gestational womb as a hazardous material and so has no objection in principle to gestational surrogacy. Weinberg, *The Risk of a Lifetime*, 245–46. It is not clear to me, however, how to draw a principled difference between gametes and the gestational womb such that the first, but not the second, counts as a hazardous material (from the point of view of procreation). This observation points to a real challenge to the Hazmat Theory, namely that it won't be able to rule out, in a principled way, *any* (or at least very many) of the causal contributions to procreation as hazardous material and so fall prey to the "too many parents" objection to the causal theories of parenthood. In response, Weinberg has suggested to me that gametes—and not wombs—are the proper locus of our attention because they can grow into people. They are, in that sense, more hazardous and so demand a higher standard of care (personal correspondence).

[43] Whether actual parental responsibilities can be transferred depends on what you think those responsibilities are. See above (p. 164).

is conception. The reality, though, is that neither donors nor recipients have any interest in waiting until then to settle matters of parental responsibility. So the real question is: How early can prospective parental responsibilities be transferred?

The answer is: at least as early as the time of donation. Indeed, the two events—provision of the gametes and transfer of prospective parental responsibilities—can come as a package. I imagine this is exactly as donors and recipients—at least in the case of personal donation—want it. Having provided the gametes, the donor is no longer responsible for their care or, more generally, on the hook for living up to the demands of prospective parental responsibility. Contrariwise, the recipients incur full prospective parental responsibility. They are not beholden to the demands or wishes of the donor with respect to how the gametes are used.

The "how" and "when" of transfer are more complicated when it comes to impersonal donation. With impersonal donation the donor does not pick out the recipients. Instead, an intermediary—a sperm or egg clinic—does. Moreover, this intermediary typically holds onto the gametes for a time (sometimes, a very long time) between donation and provision. Assume now that the intermediary is effective at picking out adequate intended parents. When does the transfer of prospective parental responsibilities take place? And to whom? Does the intermediary become prospectively parentally responsible at any point?

I don't think there is any single morally mandated answer to these questions. The goal, recall, is to get parental responsibility from the person who doesn't want it (the donor) to the people who want it (the prospective parents). This goal is consistent with the donor transferring prospective parental responsibilities to the intermediary at the time of donation and then having the intermediary transfer prospective parental responsibilities to the prospective parents at the time of gamete provision. But it is also consistent with the donor retaining prospective parental responsibilities until the point of gamete provision. The donor, in this case, would *delegate* the responsibilities of prospective parental responsibilities to the intermediary without, in fact giving, them up.

The distinction between transferring versus delegating prospective parental responsibilities is not merely semantic.[44] For in the case of delegation,

---

[44] The distinction between delegating and transferring parental responsibilities is made by Reuven Brandt, "The Transfer and Delegation of Responsibilities for Genetic Offspring in Gamete Provision," *Journal of Applied Philosophy* 34, no. 5 (2017): 665–78.

but not transfer, the donor retains the right to "withdraw" the gametes from circulation (in just the same way that "traditional" intended parents might decide to *stop* trying to conceive a child). But they also retain ultimate responsibility for care of the gametes as well as whether the transfer of prospective parenthood to the intended parents is responsibly done.

Figuring out whether there is reason to prefer one system over the other—as a donor, as an intermediary, as an intended parent and, finally, as a society—is a complex policy issue that I won't attempt to adjudicate. The central point is just that the presence of an intermediary poses no insuperable difficulties for answering questions about how, when, and to whom prospective parental responsibilities is transferred. There are options.

5. Do donors have a duty to be open donors?

Here's where we are. Gamete donors become prospective parents in donating. But prospective parenthood can be permissibly transferred. So, gamete donation is not, on its own, morally objectionable.[45] We know, however, that conceiving children with *anonymously* donated gametes is, normally, wrong.[46] My argument for that conclusion focused entirely on the intended parents, the people who *use* anonymously donated gametes to conceive a child. But we might wonder whether the donor bears any responsibility here. Do potential donors have any responsibility to choose to be open donors rather than anonymous donors?

They do. I offer two very closely related arguments for this conclusion. The first appeals to an idea from chapter 1, namely the principle of procreative beneficence. That principle, you'll recall, says that if we have choices about the kind of people we create, we have a weighty reason to create the people whose lives will go best.[47] This principle, combined with the Significant Interest view, enjoins people who plan to conceive with donated gametes to use an

---

[45] At least from the point of view of what parental responsibility demands.

[46] Again, on the assumption that one has a choice between using an anonymous and an open donor.

[47] This is a simplified version of what Kahane and Savulescu call the *Principle of Procreative Beneficence*:

> If couples (or single reproducers) have decided to have a child and selection is possible, then they have a significant moral reason to select the child, of the possible children they could have, whose life can be expected, in light of the relevant available information, to go best or [at] least not worse than any of the others.

Julian Savulescu and Guy Kahane, "The Moral Obligation to Create Children with the Best Chance of the Best Life," *Bioethics* 23, no. 5 (2009): 274.

open donor. But it also gives prospective donors a weighty reason to be open donors. For while donors will not be normative parents, they are still making choices about what kinds of people will come into existence, namely people who will or will not have access to genetic knowledge. Inasmuch as there is reason to think that it is generally good (overall) for a donor-conceived person to have access to genetic knowledge, then the principle of procreative beneficence tells us that prospective donors—as procreators—have a weighty moral reason to be open donors.[48]

The second argument for why donors should be open donors appeals to a more general claim about participating in a morally problematic practice. The idea is this: if conceiving a child with an anonymous donor is (usually) morally unacceptable, then providing gametes for the purpose of conceiving a child with an anonymous donor is (usually) morally unacceptable. To put it more simply, if intended parents shouldn't be using anonymous gametes, then donors should not be contributing to efforts to use anonymously donated gametes. The reason is perfectly general: if doing something is wrong, then intentionally helping someone do that thing is also at least presumptively wrong.

Crucially, my claim is *not* that the intended parents will be bad parents. I have already claimed that that is unlikely to be true, or at least no more likely to be true than it is with "traditional" parents. They might well be wonderful parents: loving, warm, generous, *etc.* Using an anonymous donor is a parental failure, but it does not constitute a *gross* dereliction of parental duty. Nor is it evidence for overall parental inadequacy. So my claim is not that anonymous donors are giving gametes to people who will be bad parents. Even so, conceiving with anonymously donated gametes is (usually) a parental failure, and not an insignificant one if the argument of the first part of the book is correct. Intended parents who prefer to conceive with anonymously donated gametes are doing something they shouldn't. And so, a donor who donates anonymously in order to meet the need of these intended parents is intentionally implicating themselves in a morally impermissible practice.

Both arguments leave open the possibility that, *all things considered*, it is permissible to be an anonymous donor. The principle of procreative

---

[48] Indeed, properly taking into consideration the principle of procreative beneficence is plausibly one of the duties of prospective parenthood. It is worth adding that the prospective parents have even more reason to choose an open donor owing to the specifically parental responsibility of promoting their child's well-being.

beneficence provides a weighty reason to be an open donor . . . but perhaps there are reasons to be an anonymous donor that outweigh it. Intentionally helping someone do something wrong is presumptively wrong . . . but maybe there are reasons for thinking the presumption should be withdrawn. The task is the same no matter which argument we go with: namely, to identify whether there are reasons for being an anonymous donor that outweigh the reasons in favor of being an open donor. In what follows, I'll frame things in terms of the second argument and ask whether there are reasons to be an anonymous donor that make participating in the morally problematic practice permissible. But nothing really hangs on whether we focus on one argument or the other.[49]

Here's one thing we already know: there are not *parent-focused* reasons, i.e. reasons that appeal to the interests some intended parents have in using an anonymous donor. Why? Because we already know intended parents (usually) have decisive reason to use an open donor *even given those interests*.[50] In other words, given that intended parents have decisive reason not to use an anonymous donor, prospective donors cannot justify donating anonymously by appealing to the interests of some intended parents to use an anonymous donor. We already know those interests are not weighty enough to justify the use of an anonymous donor. So, parent-focused reasons won't justify being an anonymous donor.

But perhaps there are other reasons for donating that might make participating in the morally problematic practice *all things considered* permissible. In the United States, donors are compensated for their donation. According to Rene Almeling, "[T]he vast majority of egg and sperm donors I interviewed revealed that their initial interest in donation was sparked by the prospect of financial compensation."[51] These donors' reasons for donating are not parent-focused. Rather, they are *self-focused*.

Can self-focused reasons for donating anonymously justify participating in the morally problematic practice? It depends how weighty they are. Suppose I agree to help someone bury their murder victim for $10. I have no independent interest in contributing to the murderer's morally nefarious project. I'm not doing it *for* the murderer. I'm doing it for the money (for myself). But, barring exceptional circumstances, this self-focused reason is

---

[49] On the assumption that if we find a reason that works against one of the arguments, it works against the other as well.

[50] This was the conclusion of chapter 6.

[51] Rene Almeling, *Sex Cells: The Medical Market for Eggs and Sperm* (Berkeley: University of California Press, 2011), 112.

not nearly weighty enough to justify helping the murderer. Hitmen aren't off the hook because they're only in it for the money. Suppose, though, that the safety of my family depends on my helping bury the victim. If I help, I'm still participating in an immoral act. But here we might all agree that my (self-focused) reasons for acting are so weighty that I am justified in helping.

So we need to know whether the financial reasons for donating are so weighty that they justify contributing to the morally problematic practice of conceiving children with anonymously donated gametes. The first thing to note is that financial reasons for donating gametes don't provide any reason for donating *anonymously*. In fact, the opposite is true. Being an open donor pays more than being an anonymous donor. But suppose that weren't true, and financial considerations gave potential donors a reason to be anonymous. Are those considerations weighty enough to make anonymous donation acceptable (given that one will be contributing to a morally impermissible project)?

They might be if the donor were in dire financial straits, which could be remedied by donating. Almeling notes that it is "understandable" that most donors are (at least initially) in it for the money, "given their life circumstances."[52] Most of the donors she interviewed

> [w]ere working but were doing so in low-paying jobs that were often part-time. Moreover, about half of all donors were also students, including those who were taking a few classes at the local junior college and those who were enrolled full-time at a four-year university.[53]

But Almeling's interviews make clear that the donors did not see themselves as *desperate* for the money. Rather, they saw donation as a relatively easy and morally unproblematic way to make some extra money.[54] But for reasons that are by now familiar, it is *not* morally unproblematic to anonymously donate gametes.[55] So, inasmuch as the financial reasons to donate anonymously are not exigent, it is implausible they are weighty enough to justify anonymous gamete donation.[56]

---

[52] Almeling, *Sex Cells*, 112.

[53] Almeling, *Sex Cells*, 112.

[54] Egg donors stand to make somewhere between $3,000 and $8,000 per donation. Sperm donors stand to earn anywhere from $600 to $1,200 a month if they donate regularly (about three times a week!).

[55] Not of all of Almeling's interview subjects were anonymous donors.

[56] And even if they were, the right conclusion is that anonymous donors find themselves in a morally compromised situation, one where financial pressures are so overwhelming that they are all

The conclusion is the same even if the self-focused reason for being an anonymous donor is not about money, but instead an interest in not being involved—in any way—with the resulting child. Indeed, this is what happens with donors who do it for the money but choose to donate anonymously: the money gets them through the door, but they choose anonymity for other reasons (since financial considerations alone would lead them to be open donors). But even if donating for financial reasons is not morally problematic,[57] doing so knowing that one will choose anonymity *is* and for just the reasons we've already looked at: the financial reasons to donate don't outweigh the moral reasons not to do so anonymously. Donors might have weighty reasons to choose anonymity *given* that they are donating. But they are not *forced* to donate. They choose to do so. And if they know in advance that they will choose to donate anonymously, the financial reasons are not weighty enough to justify donating (given that the donation will be anonymous). In other words, donors cannot treat the choice to donate and the choice to donate *anonymously* as two separate decisions, with the first justified by financial considerations and the second justified by the (admittedly weighty) reason that they do not want to be involved with their future genetic offspring. Rather, whether financial considerations are weighty enough to justify donating depends, in part, on whether the donation will be anonymous or not.

So neither purely parent-focused reasons nor purely self-focused reasons (of the sort that actually move people to donate) justify being an anonymous gamete donor. But what if the donor's motives are a *mix* of parent-focused and self-focused reasons? Suppose the donor's reason for donating in the first place is that they altruistically want to help people have a child who otherwise would not be able to. The intended parents' interest in having a child is the reason the donor donates. But then the reason the donor chooses to donate *anonymously* is self-focused. He doesn't want to have a connection to the resulting child. He decides to donate for altruistic reasons, but then appeals to the (weighty) self-focused reason to do so anonymously. If the donor knows he will donate anonymously, then he confronts a weighty reason not

things considered justified in contributing to a morally problematic practice. The proper solution is to remedy the situation that results in people finding themselves in the morally compromised situation and not resting content with the thought that they act permissibly in that situation.

[57] Although maybe it is! I take no stand on that issue here.

to donate at all. But in this case that reason is plausibly counterbalanced by the altruistic reason to donate.[58]

Perhaps, then, there is a general case where being an anonymous donor is permissible. Notice, though, that this case falls apart if it turns out that intended parents don't need *anonymously* donated gametes in order to have a child. If there is an adequate supply of open donors, then our imagined altruistic potential donor who wants to remain anonymous has no reason to donate.[59] But let's set that issue aside for now and consider the case where there is a need for our imagined donor's gametes. Whether we in fact have a case where being an anonymous donor is permissible depends on assessing the relative weights of (a) the intended parents' interest in conceiving a child with donated gametes, (b) the donor's interest in being anonymous, and (c) any future child's (likely) interest in knowing who the donor is.[60] But we do not need to wade into those weeds to see that it is going to be hard to make the case that a donor's interest in anonymity both outweighs the child's likely interest in knowing the donor *and* is outweighed by the parent's interest in having a child with donated gametes. Why?

Well, we know many donor-conceived people have a significant interest that is tied to identity formation. How does the donor's interest in being anonymous compare to that? It is not hard to imagine why some donors want to be anonymous. They don't want any future entanglement with the child and all the possible emotional and family-related complications that might entail. How weighty are considerations of this sort?

If we see them as something more like inconveniences—not insubstantial ones, but inconveniences nonetheless—then it seems implausible that the donor's interest in anonymity is equivalent to, let alone weightier than, the child's interest to have an open donor. But suppose it is more than an inconvenience, that it is a significant interest in its own right that can compete—as it were—with the child's interest. The problem now is that the weightier

---

[58] Some might be skeptical that there really *are* altruistic donors. But there are. Almeling notes, "About a fifth of the donors [interviewed] started out with a very different motivation: they were primarily interested in helping recipients have children. In comparison to donors who were 'in it for the money,' these donors were at a different point in their lives, more likely to be married, to have children, to be financially comfortable." Almeling, *Sex Cells*, 115.

[59] I return to the empirical question of the supply of open versus anonymous donors in chapter 8.

[60] Clearly, there are some prospective donors who, if they are convinced by my argument, will choose not to donate at all rather than be an open donor. And this may lead some to wonder whether the frustrated interest of people conceived with anonymously donated gametes should count at all given that being conceived via an anonymous donor is a condition of their existence. For my answer to this line of thought, see chapter 1.

the donor's interest in anonymity—i.e. the more important it is to the donor that they not be entangled with the future child—the more likely it is that their interest will outweigh the intended parents' interest in having a child with donated gametes. In other words, if it is *so* important to the prospective donor that he be anonymous, then he should not donate in the first place.[61]

So in order for altruistic anonymous donation to be permissible, the donor's interest in anonymity needs to be weighty enough to outweigh the child's likely future interest in having genetic knowledge but not so weighty that it outweighs the intended parents' interest in conceiving a child with donated gametes (and so gives the prospective donor decisive reason not to donate at all). Maybe the interest in anonymity can thread the needle, but it seems unlikely, *especially* if the intended parents' interest can be met by an open donor (which they should be using anyway).

This last point is important. For even if altruistic anonymous donation is permissible, that doesn't change the fact that *using* an anonymous donor when open donors are available is still (normally) impermissible. So, intended parents that prefer to use an anonymous donor cannot appeal to the permissibility of being an altruistic anonymous donor (if, indeed, it is permissible) to justify using an anonymous donor. They should use an open donor if one is available. The need for altruistic anonymous donors only arises, then, if there is an undersupply of open donors. Since intended parents ought to use an open donor, the goal, from a policy point of view, should be to ensure an adequate supply of open donors.

6. Conclusion

So here's where we are: even if gamete donation triggers parental responsibility, it does not follow that gamete donors incur parental responsibility. Rather, they become prospectively parentally responsible, a status that can be transferred even if parental responsibility cannot be. While there might be extrinsic reasons for doubting that prospective parental responsibilities can be responsibly transferred, there are no intrinsic reasons for thinking so. Moreover, the transfer can happen at the time of procurement (which happens—more or less—at the time of donation with known donation and at a later time with impersonal donation).

---

[61] All the more so given concerns about the *de facto* end of anonymity.

But even if gamete donors are parentally off the hook at, or shortly after, the time of donation, they should not be anonymous donors for the sake of helping intended parents meet their interest of conceiving with anonymously donated gametes. Some people might justifiably choose to donate for self-focused reasons, but those reasons don't justify *anonymous* donation. The only circumstances where anonymous donation might be justified are those where the donor's reasons for donating are altruistic, but the reasons for being anonymous are self-focused. Even here I have suggested it is unlikely to be permissible given the nature of the competing interests. Most importantly, none of this changes the fact that intended parents ought to avoid using anonymous donors where they can. Ideally, there would be nearly no demand for anonymous donors.

8

Policy and Practice

I have argued that intended parents who plan to use donated gametes should use an open donor. I've also argued that anyone who plans to be a donor should be an open donor. What do these conclusions mean for how donor conception systems should be run? More specifically, do they warrant the conclusion that anonymous gamete donation should be legally prohibited?

The short answer, I will argue, is "no." Even though creating children with anonymously donated gametes is (usually) morally wrong, people should be legally allowed to do it. This is partly because the failure to use an open donor is on a par with other permissible parental failures. But it is also because legally prohibiting anonymous gamete donation without simultaneously working to disrupt the bionormative schema we all inhabit will have *expressive effects*—i.e. effects that express some idea or commitment—that we should avoid. This last point leads to a longer answer to the question of whether anonymous gamete donation should be prohibited: if legal prohibition should be pursued, it should only happen in the context of combating our culture's bionormativity so as to minimize the expressive effects of simply outlawing anonymous gamete donation.

In light of this longer answer, I identify three representative "levels" at which the bionormative schema should be disrupted: the legal level, the educational level, and the personal level. I offer nothing like a thoroughgoing vision for how to revamp practices and policies at these levels. That is beyond my ken. Instead, I point to examples, some of which we encountered in previous chapters, of the kinds of things we should aim to change as part of a broader move to make open donation the legal norm.

I conclude by returning to an issue I raised in the first chapter. The central point of this book has been to show that intended parents should use an open donor. But some might wonder whether my arguments establish that intended parents should use a *known* donor rather than an open donor. I will suggest—and truly only suggest—that my arguments might support this stronger conclusion. Using a known donor introduces complications

Conceiving People. Daniel Groll, Oxford University Press. © Oxford University Press 2021.
DOI: 10.1003/oso/9780100063054.003.0008

that block the conclusion that, in general, intended parents should use a known donor.

1. Should anonymous donation be legally prohibited?

In a way, the horse has already left the barn. Anonymous donation is already legally prohibited in a good number of places and there is no realistic prospect things will change. There are places where it is permitted, including the United States and Canada. But even in those places, the legal issue is less pressing than it once was for reasons I talked about in the first chapter. The availability of cheap DNA testing combined with the powers of the internet means that no one who donates should be at all confident their identity will remain unknown. Moreover, there is a move toward openness in donor conception. For example, the California Cryobank, the largest gamete clinic in the United States, "has stopped offering anonymity to its new donors. Donors now must agree to reveal their names to their offspring when they turn 18 and to have some form of communication to be mediated, at first, by the bank."[1] So, it could be that in years to come the practice of anonymous donation becomes a thing of the past without any legal remedy.

But we are certainly not there now in the United States and Canada. There is a big difference between anonymous donation being less common than it once was and it disappearing altogether. And there is a big difference between the possibility of "unofficially" tracking down the identity of a donor who wanted to remain anonymous and having guaranteed access to the identity of a donor who is willing to be identified. Part of the difference is numerical, so to speak: while it is increasingly common to discover the identity of an anonymous donor, it is by no means a sure thing. So, being content with the idea that it is increasingly easy to discover a donor's identity will still leave a large number of donor-conceived people in the dark. But there is also a moral difference between a system that puts the work of discovery on the shoulders of donor-conceived people (who must wrestle with difficult questions about tracking down a genetic parent who wished to remain anonymous) and a system that ensures anyone who donates is willing, and able, to be identified.

---

[1] Susan Dominus, "Sperm Donors Can't Stay Secret Anymore: Here's What That Means," *New York Times*, June 26, 2019, https://www.nytimes.com/2019/06/26/magazine/sperm-donor-questions. html.

For all these reasons, the legal question is hardly irrelevant even in an age when donors can no longer have confidence they will remain anonymous. So, should anonymous gamete donation be legally prohibited?

1.1. One argument against prohibiting anonymous donation

One argument for allowing anonymous gamete donation combines a practical worry with a claim about justice. The practical worry is that there will be a shortage of donors if anonymous donation is prohibited. This concern is somewhat borne out by the data. Godman et al. report that in Western Australia, where all donation has been open donation since December 2004, "the total number of sperm donors . . . has halved and the recruitment of new donors declined by ~32%."[2] In the Netherlands, "[d]uring 15 years of debate on the abolition of donor anonymity the number of donors decreased by >70% and the number of semen banks by 50%."[3] In the UK, where donor anonymity was outlawed in 2004, it is generally acknowledged that "there are now too few donors coming forward to provide all patients who need sperm donor-assisted conception with treatment."[4]

The claim about justice is that denying people the chance to start a family with donated gametes is unjust. This line of thought is strengthened by the fact that a substantial subset of the people for whom this is an issue—namely LGBTQ+ people—are members of groups that are marginalized partly and precisely because they buck norms and expectations about what families should look like. Preventing such people from having children by scuttling the supply of available gametes has the effect of reinforcing this marginalization ("Family-making is not for you!") even if that is not the intent of the policy. In light of this, there is a strong reason not to make anonymous donation illegal.

In order to make this argument convincing, a lot more would need to be said about both the practical claim and the justice claim. With respect to the

[2] Kate M. Godman et al., "Potential Sperm Donors', Recipients' and Their Partners' Opinions towards the Release of Identifying Information in Western Australia," *Human Reproduction* 21, no. 11 (2006): 3022.

[3] P. M. W. Janssens et al., "A New Dutch Law Regulating Provision of Identifying Information of Donors to Offspring: Background, Content and Impact," *Human Reproduction* 21, no. 4 (2006): 852.

[4] Allan Pacey, "Sperm Donor Recruitment in the UK," *Obstetrician & Gynaecologist* 12, no. 1 (2010): 47. See also Madhavi Gudipati et al., "The Sperm Donor Programme over 11 Years at Newcastle Fertility Centre," *Human Fertility* 16, no. 4 (2013): 258–65.

first, there appears to be a strong correlation between outlawing anonymity and a reduced number of donors. But it is not clear whether the decline in the number of donors reflects a fundamental unwillingness of people to be open donors (and so is largely irremediable) or instead reflects the ineffectiveness of traditional recruitment methods.

There is some evidence it is the latter. Dr. Kamal Ahuja, the Scientific and Managing Director of the London Sperm Bank, reported in 2015, "For the first time, a British sperm bank—the London Sperm Bank (LSB)—has sufficient stocks and donors to begin supplying clinics registered with the Human Fertilisation and Embryology Authority (HFEA). The move marks a shift in the dynamics of UK sperm donation."[5] He attributes the dramatic increase in supply to "an alternative and innovative approach to donor recruitment, with amplified modern communication tools and personalised customer care to reach and encourage a wider pool of responders."[6] The lesson, then, might be that we can have our cake and eat it too: anonymous donation can be outlawed *and* there can be an adequate supply of domestic donors.[7]

What about the second claim, namely that denying people the chance to start a family with donated gametes is unjust: Is that true? To show that it is, we would need an account of why justice demands the opportunity to start a family *via* gamete donation when adoption is also an option. Granted, it is not an easy option for all kinds of reasons.[8] But it is an option. If there are people who want to be parents but cannot conceive children with their own gametes, then justice might demand that they be given an opportunity to start a family in some other way, but that other way need not be *via* donor conception. We would need a further argument to get the conclusion that justice demands the latter.[9]

---

[5] Kamal K. Ahuja, "Is the UK Sperm Donor Shortage a Myth?," *BioNews*, May 2015, https://www. bionews.org.uk/page_95041.

[6] Ahuja, "Is the UK Sperm Donor Shortage a Myth?"

[7] On the other hand, there is a shortage of donors in Sweden, which has had more than 30 years to work out an effective donor recruitment strategy. And there is no shortage in Norway, where all donation is anonymous (and where intended parents from countries that don't allow anonymous donation travel to procure sperm). See Erling Ekerhovd and Anders Faurskov, "Swedish Sperm Donors Are Driven by Altruism, but Shortage of Sperm Donors Leads to Reproductive Travelling," *Upsala Journal of Medical Sciences* 113, no. 3 (2008): 305–14.

[8] This first-person account powerfully spells out some of them: Farai Chideya, "Excuse Me, May I Raise Your Child?," *Medium*, July 8, 2019, https://zora.medium.com/ excuse-me-may-i-raise-your-child-45afc26f088d.

[9] The question of whether the state should fund fertility treatment has been extensively discussed. It is not the same issue as that raised above, but some of the considerations are much the same. For an argument that the state should not fund fertility treatment except for same-sex couples, see Emily McTernan, "Should Fertility Treatment Be State Funded?," *Journal of Applied Philosophy* 32, no. 3 (2015): 227–40. McTernan's article also has a great list of articles on this topic.

Perhaps that further argument could go through intended parents' specific interest in having a child that is genetically related to at least one of them. You can't get that *via* adoption.[10] But now the question is whether the interest in conceiving and raising a genetic child is weighty enough to get us to the conclusion that justice demands people be permitted to conceive a genetic child with anonymously donated gametes (assuming that the supply of open donors is inadequate to meet demand).

Rather than directly tackle that question, we can return to an earlier point: there is likely to be a symmetry between an account of the importance of conceiving and raising one's genetic child and an account of the significance of genetic knowledge to a donor-conceived person. That is, a case for conceiving and raising one's genetic child that appeals to the profound importance of genetic relatedness for childrearing[11] will simultaneously lend support to an account of the importance of genetic relatedness *for the child*.[12] So, we are likely to end up with something close to a "tie" between the weighty parental interest in conceiving with anonymously donated gametes[13] and the child's interest in being conceived with an open donor.

Now, maybe a careful account of the situation will show that things tilt in favor of the intended parents.[14] The point I'm making here is just that a strategy for defending the legal permissibility of anonymous donation that combines practical considerations—about the supply of open versus anonymous donors—with arguments about the justice of conceiving and raising one's own genetic children is hardly a slam dunk. Moreover, it may well need to appeal (however implicitly) to a premise about the profound importance of genetic ties, which would serve to also undermine the argument for allowing anonymous donation.

---

[10] Except in exceptional circumstances, such as adopting a sibling's child should your sibling die or be unable to care for their child. Thanks to Dorothy McKinnon for pointing this out.

[11] An account I obviously reject.

[12] Likewise, an account of the relative unimportance of genetic relatedness for children will simultaneously lend support to the relative unimportance for parents of conceiving and rearing genetically related children and so be less likely to ground the claim that justice demands that people be given the opportunity to conceive and raise genetic children.

[13] Assuming, as we are, that this is the only way of meeting the interest in conceiving a genetic child.

[14] Or maybe there is a parent-centered rationale for conceiving with a donor that does not imply a symmetrical reason for a child having genetic knowledge. For example, someone might ground an interest in conceiving with a donor in an interest in being pregnant and birthing a child.

2. The Parity argument

Is there another way to defend the conclusion that anonymous donation should be legally permitted? I think there is. The account I prefer depends on two ideas. First, parents rightly have wide legal discretion *to parentally fail* in various respects. Second, the parental failure involved in using an anonymous donor is exactly the kind of parental failure that the state should allow.

I doubt anyone seriously doubts the first claim. But it is worth being clear about what exactly it means, particularly in light of a cultural presumption that parents should *always* act in their children's best interest. A moment's thought exposes that presumption as false. Indeed, in many cases, parents are morally required to act contrary to their child's best interests. Consider two examples from Matthew Clayton, one about intentionally harming others and the other about foreseeably doing so in order to benefit his child:

> Although my child's wellbeing might be improved if I kidnapped an effective mathematics tutor or cricket coach and forced her to perfect my child's arithmetic or spin bowling, I am not morally permitted to do so. [. . .] Suppose that taking my child for a walk in the woods to enhance her understanding of the natural world would foreseeably release hundreds of wasps that would inflict harm on other people near the wood. If the harm done to others were disproportionate, I would not be permitted to improve my child's wellbeing in that way.[15]

To put the point simply: justice limits what people may do for the good of their children.

Usually, however, when people talk about doing what is best for their child, they mean that they will do so within the bounds of justice (or at least without stepping wildly outside those bounds). Just what those bounds are is none too clear. Conventional understandings of the bounds of justice—which allow well-to-do parents to confer all kinds of advantages on their children—probably don't track the actual bounds of justice.[16] But let's set

---

[15] Matthew Clayton, "Anti-Perfectionist Childrearing," in *The Nature of Children's Well-Being*, ed. Alexander Bagattini and Colin Macleod (New York: Springer, 2015), 123–24. Clayton also points to a third possible source of prohibitions to acting for one's child's best interests: you might have duties to yourself that disallow you from, for example, selling yourself into slavery for the sake of your child.

[16] Harry Brighouse and Adam Swift, *Family Values: The Ethics of Parent-Child Relationships* (Princeton, NJ: Princeton University Press, 2014), chapter 5; Colin MacLeod, "Parental Responsibilities in an Unjust World," in *Procreation and Parenthood: The Ethics of Bearing and*

those worries aside for now, and consider the idea that within the bounds of justice, parents ought always to do what is best for their children.

Now, if by "children" we mean children at any age, the idea is almost certainly false. Once a child has reached adulthood, a parent's pursuit of the child's good is properly constrained by the child's autonomy, i.e. their right to make decisions about their own life. A parent who acts against an adult child's wishes is acting in an unduly paternalistic manner. So, a parent's pursuit of their child's good is constrained by demands of justice and the child's autonomy when she is autonomous.[17]

But suppose we are limiting ourselves to young children and we have taken on board the demands of justice. Surely now it is true that parents must act in the best interests of their child. Not so fast. Parents are people too. They have their own projects and interests. It is not crazy to think that parents may, at least sometimes, subordinate the interests of their children to their own. Suppose a parent's dream job requires putting his child in a slightly worse, but still good school. It is not crazy to think that the parent can do this, particularly if we imagine that he finds his current work dissatisfying.[18]

It is always possible to spin stories according to which decisions like this are really in the child's best interest, e.g. a parent who is satisfied at work will be a better parent at home. There is something to these stories; they reflect what I call the "oxygen mask" model of thinking about family interests. Taking care of yourself (putting on your oxygen mask first) better enables you to take care of the people in your charge.[19] But they can easily be just-so stories. A decision that, on the face of it, was made *for* the parent gets justified in terms of the best interest of the child. It is more reasonable, I think, to acknowledge that good parents sometimes act in their own interests over their child's ("Yes, you can watch another TV show. Please let me sleep!") and that they don't do anything wrong in doing so. If that's true, then even within the

---

Rearing Children, ed. David Archard and David Benatar (New York: Oxford University Press, 2010), 128–150.

[17] It also constrained, in some way, by the need to respect their *future* autonomy. But just how it is constrained is unclear. On my skepticism about the autonomy route settling the central issue of this book, see chapter 1 and chapter 3.

[18] For a critique of the ethos of "intensive" parenting that might make this decision seem unacceptable to many parents, see Joan C. Tronto, "The 'Nanny' Question in Feminism," *Hypatia* 17, no. 2 (2002): 35. Tronto speaks specifically of the demands of intensive *mothering*, a concept she gets from Sharon Hays, *The Cultural Contradictions of Motherhood* (New Haven, CT: Yale University Press, 1996), preface x.

[19] Daniel Groll, "Four Models of Family Interests," *Pediatrics* 134, Supplement 2 (2014): S82.

constraints of justice and autonomy, parents needn't always do what is best for their child.

Clearly, not acting in your child's best interest should be legal when morality demands it or when parental self-interest permits it. But I don't want to focus on these ways of not acting in your child's best interest. Instead, my focus will be on *failing* to act in your child's best interest, where that means *not acting in your child's best interest when you should*. To put it differently, not acting in your child's best interest when doing so is contrary to morality or permitted by parental self-interest is *not* a failure to act in your child's best interest in the sense I intend.[20] When I speak of parental failure, I mean to pick out things that parents do that, all things considered, they shouldn't do *as* parents.

It is not unreasonable to wonder whether parental *failures* should be subject to legal sanction. Some obviously should be. Parental failures that seriously threaten the safety and well-being of children are rightly outlawed. But equally obviously, others should not be. Parents make mistakes, or fail, their children all the time. A confession: I routinely raise my voice when my daughter is practicing piano. This is a parental failure, but not one that should be sanctioned by the law. We have a range of parental failures, then, from severe (e.g. abuse) to very minor (losing patience while supervising piano practice).

Using an anonymous donor is not a trivial parental failure. Donor-conceived children are likely to have a significant interest in obtaining genetic knowledge, an interest that is often bound up with identity determination. Intentionally putting them in a position where that interest is likely to be frustrated is a significant parental failure. But it is not *severe* if that term is reserved for parental failures that seriously threaten the safety and well-being of the child. Indeed, it is of a piece with all kinds of other parental failures that are not sanctioned by the law. Parents can (and often do) profoundly affect their children in ways that they shouldn't. Think about all the things that parents routinely fail to do for their children: read to them; save for their education; feed them healthy food on a regular basis; give them enough sleep; not yell at them angrily for some small infraction; not pass on their own neuroses about weight or masculinity or money. The list goes on and on!

To put it bluntly, parents have wide latitude to mess up their kids. The decision to use an anonymous donor is, at worst, just another instance of parental

---

[20] I'm not saying you couldn't use the term for those contexts. Only that I am not using it for them.

failure of this kind. Presumptively, then, it should be treated the same way: if the other examples of parental failure are not subject to legal sanction, then neither should *this* particular parental failure. I call this the Parity argument.

One response to the Parity argument grants that all these cases of significant parental failure should be treated the same from a legal point of view. But it claims that rather than conclude that *none* of them should be legally sanctioned, we should conclude that *all* of them should be.

I assume no one would advocate for this view. Seeing why, however, points to a considerably more compelling response to the Parity argument. For suppose we ask: Why should parents be given wide legal discretion to fail their children? At least part of the answer is that the cure would be worse than the disease. Any legal system that sanctioned significant but, frankly, run-of-the-mill parental failures like those above would create more (serious) problems than it solves. Legal mechanisms that were effective in preventing the kinds of parental failures we're talking about would likely be extraordinarily intrusive. The government would have considerable power to dictate how families function. Such a state of affairs would be worrying even if the government were perfect executors of the laws we're now imagining (i.e. targeting only those people that should be targeted and doing so in the right way). But it becomes profoundly worrying when we acknowledge that the government is not a perfect executor of the law. Even when it is well intentioned, mistakes will be made. And then it becomes utterly terrifying when we acknowledge that the government is often *not* a well-intentioned executor of the law, both in general and with respect to family-related law.[21]

The line of thought is inspired by John Stuart Mill's account of justice and its relation to morality. Mill claimed that morality is about bringing about the best consequences. For Mill, the quality of consequences is a function of how much overall happiness they produce. So, for Mill, the *morally best* action in any given situation is the one that produces the most overall happiness. Mill recognized, however, that there are all kinds of actions that, while not the best they could be morally speaking, should nonetheless be treated as morally acceptable. In other words, Mill recognized that an adequate moral system, and in particular acceptable practices of holding others and ourselves morally accountable, needs to leave space for actions that, while not the very best they

---

[21] See Laura Briggs, *Somebody's Children: The Politics of Transracial and Transnational Adoption* (Durham, NC: Duke University Press, 2012), part 1. See also Annette Appell, "The Endurance of Biological Connection: Heteronormativity, Same-Sex Parenting and the Lessons of Adoption," *BYU Journal of Public Law* 22, no. 2 (2008): 294–97.

could be, are still morally acceptable. Why does an adequate moral theory need to leave this kind of space? For Mill, the reason was simple: doing otherwise would make things worse overall.[22] Society would end up intruding on the lives of people in a way that would make things worse overall.

We don't need to sign on to Mill's moral theory to sign on to this last thought. Every reader can think of a situation where there was no way to right a wrong, to correct a mistake, to send someone down the right path, without making things worse. We often confront situations where the best thing to do is let someone fail because there is no way to step in without making things worse, either in the case at hand or by setting a terrible precedent. In general, parental failures of the kind we're thinking about are examples of this sort. There is no way for the government to legally sanction them—in a way that would effectively prevent them from happening—without making the situation for families (including the children we are aiming to protect) worse overall.

What does this have to do with the Parity argument? The idea is that even if it is true *in general* that trying to prevent parental failures of the kind we're talking about would make things worse overall, the parental failure of conceiving a child with anonymously donated gametes is an exception. For unlike with so many of the other significant parental failures mentioned above, there is an easy and non-intrusive way to prevent the failure: simply don't allow people to donate anonymously.

The fact that basically all conception with anonymously donated gametes involves a third party—a clinic that collects and then disburses the gametes—presents the government with a convenient choke-point for non-intrusive regulation. Unlike the other parental failures mentioned above, where the government would need to have some way to monitor the goings-on in family life, *this* parental failure can be easily prevented by removing the option that allows for the failure in the first place. For this particular parental failure, then, the Millian framework suggests that a legal remedy is justified. It gets the result we're after without introducing costs that make things worse overall.

---

[22] John Stuart Mill, *Utilitarianism: And the 1868 Speech on Capital Punishment*, Hackett Classics (Indianapolis, IN: Hackett, 2002), 48–49, 54. Mill's thought was that they should not even be the subject of *moral* sanction in the form of blame or ostracization or guilt. I think he's right about that too, at least with respect to many less than fully optimal actions, but I am using his idea to make a point about legal sanctions.

It is true that the presence of the third party in the reproductive process gives the government an opportunity for an "easy" intervention, one that doesn't come with the kinds of costs involved in preventing other parental failures of the same magnitude. But that doesn't settle the matter for two reasons.

The first is that preventing anonymous donation will not, on its own, accomplish the intended goal. As we know from chapter 2, although there is increasing openness when it comes to donor conception, a very substantial portion of parents do not tell their children they were donor-conceived. If the goal is to ensure, as best as possible, that donor-conceived people really get access to genetic information, then what's really required is preventing anonymous donation *and* requiring disclosure. So perhaps the latter should be legally mandated as well. It could be accomplished "by adding to birth certificates the words 'by donation' by the father's and/or the mother's names, or by issuing a 'donor conception certificate' that would be attached to the child's birth certificate."[23]

What should we make of this package of proposed remedies of legally prohibiting anonymous donation and legally requiring disclosure? One thing to note is that the relative unobtrusiveness of prohibiting anonymous donation is somewhat undercut by also requiring disclosure. Part of why prohibiting the use of anonymously donated gametes is relatively unobtrusive is that it does not, by itself, constrain subsequent parenting. It makes available—in effect, it preserves—information for the child, but it does not mandate the provision of that information. If, however, the mandate against anonymous donation is wed to a legal requirement to disclose, then the choice to conceive with donated gametes does constrain subsequent parenting. Parents have a deadline looming. Disclosure is coming. And the fact that it is coming—one way or the other—forces an item onto the parenting agenda that might not otherwise be there (even if it should be there).

"Yes," says the proponent of legally mandated disclosure, "that is the point!" But notice that what initially looked like a relatively straightforward Millian justification for prohibiting anonymous donation—namely, that it could be done without significantly impinging on family functioning—is

---

[23] Vardit Ravitsky, "Knowing Where You Come from: The Rights of Donor-Conceived Individuals and the Meaning of Genetic Relatedness," *Minnesota Journal of Law, Science & Technology* 11 (2010): 683. Crucially, this is not Ravitsky's position, but one that she considers only to reject. She cites the following as an instance of the view: David Gollancz, "Time to Stop Lying," *Guardian*, August 2, 2007, https://www.theguardian.com/society/2007/aug/02/childrensservices.humanrights.

not so straightforward. The effectiveness of prohibiting anonymous donation depends on another requirement that certainly will impact family functioning (by forcing a conversation that parents may not want to have).

Maybe the package of requirements—mandating disclosure and
prohibiting anonymous donation—will pass the Millian test as well. But it
is hardly obvious that it will, particularly when we consider the *expressive*
effects of the package. For the position we're now considering singles out for
legal attention a portion of the population that is already considerably more
burdened than traditional intended parents when it comes to procreating.
The law says to *this* subset of intended parents what it does not say to other
parents, namely: "This particular kind of parental failure must be prevented."
Traditional parents are given wider discretion to parentally fail than non-
traditional parents.

This is especially worrying against the backdrop of bionormative prejudice that we explored back in chapter 5. The bionormative prejudice
downgrades non-traditional family forms precisely because they lack the
"full" genetic connectedness of traditional families. Consider legal mandates
to use an open donor and to disclose in this context. Such mandates will naturally be read as an attempt to provide a version of the very thing—genetic
connectedness—that, according to the bionormative prejudice, makes a
family with a donor-conceived child less than ideal. In other words, against
the backdrop of a bionormative society, the mandates will unavoidably express support for, and thereby reinforce, bionormative prejudice.

This is all the more true given the actual justification some advocates give
in support of the mandates. Consider, for example, the rationale for mandated disclosure offered by David Gollancz, who at age 12 found out he was
donor-conceived. Gollancz appeals to many of the ideas we talked about
back in chapter 4 about the importance of being able to tell a story in answer
to the question "Who am I?" in order to find one's place in the world:

> We use [stories], on every level, as a means of explaining and exploring who
> we are. I have come to believe that this storytelling is at the heart of our hu-
> manity: that it is at the heart of our ability to feel part of the world. Without
> it, we are flotsam: mere accidental concatenations of unaccountable desires
> and meaningless memories floating in the random currents of experience
> without context.[24]

---

[24] Gollancz, "Time to Stop Lying."

So far so good. But according to Gollancz, the *genetic* strand in our stories occupies a special place by, in effect, telling us what is *real* about us. Learning that he was donor-conceived meant that, in his view, he was

> [n]ot the descendant of Polish Jewish rabbis and scholars; not, in fact, cousin to my cousins or even, it seemed, properly entitled to my name.[25]

Gollancz here implicitly appeals to a biogenetic conception of family related-ness. He claims his cousins are not really his cousins and that his father's last name is not properly (is not *really*) his (as though family names were passed down via genetics!). And then he makes explicit what was only implicit:

> Of course, the sentimentalists say, "But of course you are entitled to your name, of course the culture and background of your paternal family belongs to you"—and of course they are not entirely wrong; those things can be claimed (and recently I went for the first time to Golancz, in Poland, in pre-cisely such an act of reclamation)—*but it is not the same. Being entitled to choose to claim a family heritage is not the same as simply owning it.*[26]

A little later he notes that his relationship with his father "was forever sub-ject to a sort of conditionality, *a sense of choice that does not exist between my daughters and me.*"[27] The picture we get is that the unchosen genetic tie—"the book in which half the recipe for a new human being is written"—is the thing that is *really* owned and establishes the truest, tightest connection be-tween parents and child.

This rationale for mandated disclosure is a clear instance of what I called genetic chauvinism (back in chapter 4). And insofar as this way of thinking is prevalent in society, a legal mandate to disclose will naturally be read as being "based on the most far-reaching understanding of genetic re-latedness, seeing it as a powerful connection that is embedded in the na-ture of being human."[28] And such a reading would, in fact, be right if the advocates for the mandate share Gollancz's thoughts about the importance of disclosure.

---

[25] Gollancz, "Time to Stop Lying."
[26] Gollancz, "Time to Stop Lying," emphasis added.
[27] Gollancz, "Time to Stop Lying," emphasis added.
[28] Ravitsky, "Knowing Where You Come from," 683.

The upshot is that even if there is, in principle, a rationale for mandating open donation and disclosure that does not appeal—implicitly or otherwise—to unwarranted biogenetic commitments, the *effect* of implementing such a policy will be to express support for, and so further reinforce, the biogenetic prejudice. Parents whose credentials as "real" parents are already questioned by society—precisely because they do not exemplify the full genetic relatedness of "traditional" families—would be singled out for legal attention concerning a matter that is *about the very thing that makes people question their status as (ideal) parents in the first place*. Even if the legal mandate were not the product of biogenetic prejudice, it almost certainly would have the effect of reinforcing it.

This is a substantial potential cost, one that was left out of the Millian response to the Parity argument. In my view, it tips the scale against legal mandates requiring open donation and disclosure (as a package). For recall, the goal of such moves is to prevent parental failures that, while serious, are no more serious than all kinds of other parental failures that the law allows. Given their expressive power, implementing legal remedies for these particular parental failures targets parents who are already subject to problematic attitudes about parenthood. For this reason, we should reject the package view.

Maybe the lesson here is that we should separate out the potential parental failures—the failure to use an open donor and the failure to disclose—and focus simply on the first as a target for a legal remedy. If intended parents cannot use an anonymous donor but are not legally required to disclose, then legally preventing them from using an anonymous donor would not be as burdensome as it would be when there is an additional legal requirement to disclose.

It is true that not forcing disclosure would, to some extent, undercut the purpose of making people use an open donor. But it would not entirely undermine it. For starters, it would prevent one form of deception, namely informing a child that they are donor-conceived, but that the donor was anonymous. If anonymous donation is not permitted, then learning that one is donor-conceived would imply that genetic knowledge is there for the taking.[29] It might also help parents who intend to disclose to follow through on their intention. Why? One reason parents who have used an anonymous

---

[29] Assuming the parents did not procure anonymously donated gametes from abroad and that the child knows that there is no anonymous donation where they live. Setting that point aside, we might worry that the point in this paragraph cuts both ways. If disclosing effectively comes with genetic knowledge (or the possibility of getting genetic knowledge), then parents who *otherwise* might have disclosed may decide not to. That is, given that under the scenario we're now imagining there is no real possibility of disclosing *and* preventing the child from obtaining genetic knowledge, we might worry that rates of disclosure may go down. This concern does not appear to be borne out in the available data. In the UK and Sweden, disclosure rates increased after mandated use of open

donor cite for not disclosing despite intending to is that they will not be able to answer the inevitable question: "If you are not my biological parent, then who is?"[30] But if they have used an open donor then this roadblock to following through on the intention to disclose disappears.

We might worry about the expressive effects even with this more modest proposal (i.e. mandating open donation, but not requiring disclosure). For even if parents are left to use their own judgment about whether (and how) to disclose, requiring open donation will naturally be read as an endorsement of the (purported) profound importance of genetic ties. So, we need to consider, once again, whether that cost is one worth bearing.

In thinking through that issue, we need to be aware of the differential burden the more modest proposal will impose on different people seeking to conceive with donated gametes. Decoupling the requirement to use an open donor from a further requirement to disclose only renders the requirement to use an open donor less burdensome for intended parents whose family form doesn't effectively require disclosure. As we know, disclosure rates among lesbian and single mothers is far higher than it is among heteronormative parents for the simple reason that the former's family structure effectively forces them to disclose. For non-heteronormative families, then, there is practically speaking no difference between a requirement to use an open donor with or without a further requirement to disclose.

This means that worries about further entrenching bionormative prejudice apply just as much with the more modest proposal as they did when we considered the package view. In fact, they may be even more salient here, since the families that will foreseeably be subject to the greatest burden

---

donation, although (a) not significantly and (b) the data do nothing to establish a causal relationship. Indeed, it seems plausible that the forces that resulted in laws mandating open donation also work to encourage disclosure. The main point, though, is that mandating open donation does not seem to negatively impact disclosure rates (though it may be true that it may cause some people who otherwise would have disclosed to not disclose). Claes Gottlieb, Othon Lalos, and Frank Lindblad, "Disclosure of Donor Insemination to the Child: The Impact of Swedish Legislation on Couples' Attitudes," *Human Reproduction* 15, no. 9 (2000): 2052–56; Ann Lalos, Claes Gottlieb, and Othon Lalos, "Legislated Right for Donor-Insemination Children to Know Their Genetic Origin: A Study of Parental Thinking," *Human Reproduction* 22, no. 6 (2007): 1759–68; Dorothy A. Greenfeld and Susan Caruso Klock, "Disclosure Decisions among Known and Anonymous Oocyte Donation Recipients," *Fertility and Sterility* 81, no. 6 (2004): 1565–71; Tabitha Freeman et al., "Disclosure of Sperm Donation: A Comparison between Solo Mother and Two-Parent Families with Identifiable Donors," *Reproductive Biomedicine Online* 33, no. 5 (2016): 592–600.

[30] Susan Golombok, *Modern Families: Parents and Children in New Family Forms* (Cambridge: Cambridge University Press, 2015), 100.

buck the bionormative standard not only by having a child that is not genetically related to both parents, but also by being non-heteronormative.
The families that are, in effect, required to disclose are precisely those
that are already subject to greater critical scrutiny in the culture at large
for lacking a traditional mother-father pair at the head of the family. The
more modest proposal, then, imposes a heavier burden onto families that
already face greater burdens as a result of their non-heteronormative form.
Moreover, even if the more modest proposal is not *meant* to express anything about the lesser worth of these families, it could nonetheless have
such an expressive effect or at least further entrench heteronormative
prejudice. Why? Because the families that could not practically avoid the
prospect of having the donor enter into their family life at some point are
precisely those families that the culture at large is already inclined to think
are *missing* a parent. Contrariwise, the families that *can* practically avoid
the prospect of the donor entering their family life (by not disclosing) are
precisely those that the culture at large is likely to read as complete (or not
missing a parental figure).

So, the families that the more modest proposal lets off the hook are precisely those that are seen as closer to the ideal of what a family should be. As
a result, the more modest proposal threatens to reinforce *hetero*normativity
(and, less directly, bionormativity, since heterosexual couples with a donor-
conceived child can easily "pass" as a biogenetic family). Being forced to
use an open donor will reliably generate access to genetic knowledge and
the "missing parent" in precisely those families that, from the point of view
of heteronormative prejudice, need it most (i.e. families without a mother
and father). This consideration—which, as far as I know, is not voiced or acknowledged by proponents of legally mandating open donation—gives us
some reason to resist even the more modest proposal.

The arguments in this section are, admittedly, speculative since they depend on empirical conjectures about what could plausibly happen if anonymous donation were legally mandated (both with and without a requirement
to disclose). They are, to that extent, highly provisional. But that is to be expected. It would be surprising if arguments for and against legally mandated
open donation didn't depend, at least in part, on messy and hard-to-discern
truths about the world.

3. Widening the lens: mandating open donation and combating bionormativity

Worries about the expressive effects of simply banning anonymous donation return us to a central theme from chapter 5. We live in a society rife with bionormative prejudice. The problem is not that people value genetic relatedness, but that they overvalue it. Non-genetic family ties are seen as "second best" versions of the supposedly real thing. It is no surprise, given our bionormative culture, that many donor-conceived people develop an interest in genetic knowledge. But, I argued, we should not discount the interest as nothing more than a function of bionormative prejudice. Nor should we work toward it eliminating it. Rather, we should aim to diminish bionormative prejudice so that the legitimate interest in genetic knowledge can develop and manifest in a healthier manner.

We can apply that same lesson to the issue of whether anonymous donation should be legally prohibited. One of the central arguments from section 8.2 is that given our bionormative society, prohibiting anonymous donation will plausibly have oppressive expressive effects. The conclusion, though, needn't be that we should allow anonymous donation. It might instead be this: if we want to legally prohibit anonymous donation, we should aim to achieve that in a context where it will not have the problematic expressive effects. In other words, efforts to outlaw anonymous donation should aim, as part of that effort, to disrupt the bionormative schema that would give rise to the problematic effects.

But how to disrupt the bionormative schema? Needless to say, I am in no position to offer anything like an exhaustive answer. Instead, I want to point to particular examples of how bionormativity manifests in three cultural domains: law, education, and individual behavior. One could easily add other domains, but my goal is not to survey all the ways in which bionormativity penetrates our culture. Nor is it to offer a systemic account of how to confront bionormativity in these three domains. Instead, I offer some clear examples of bionormativity in the three domains by way of pointing to the kinds of changes required to disrupt the bionormative schema.

The law. In "The Nature of Parenthood," Douglas NeJaime exhaustively shows how "those who break from traditional norms of gender and sexuality—women who separate motherhood from biological ties . . . and women and men who form families with a same-sex partner—often find their parent-child relationships discounted" by the law.[31] We saw some examples of this back in chapter 5:

In Connecticut, a married different-sex couple had a child through surrogacy and raised the child together for fourteen years. When they divorced, the court deemed the mother, who had neither a gestational nor genetic connection to the child, a legal stranger to her child. In Florida, an unmarried same-sex couple used the same donor sperm to have four children, with each woman giving birth to two children. They raised the children together until their relationship ended several years later, at which point the court left each woman with parental rights only to her two biological children. In New Jersey, a male same-sex couple used a donor egg to have a child through a gestational surrogate. The court recognized the gestational surrogate, rather than the biological father's husband (and the child's primary caretaker), as the second parent.[32]

Two more clear examples of bionormativity at work in the law—and how it can be changed—both come from Ontario, Canada.[33] Prior to 2006, lesbian couples could not record both mothers on the Statement of Live Birth, the document required to obtain a birth certificate. Four lesbian women—whose children were conceived with anonymous donors—successfully challenged the law, which now allows both mothers to be listed on the Statement of Live Birth.[34]

---

[31] Douglas NeJaime, "The Nature of Parenthood," *Yale Law Journal* 126, no. 8 (2017): 2265–66.

[32] NeJaime, "The Nature of Parenthood," 2265. The Connecticut example is Doe v. Doe, 710 A.2d 1297 (Conn. 1998). The Florida example is Russell v Pasik, 178 So. 3d 59–60 (Fla. Dist. Ct. App. 2015). The New Jersey example is A.G.R. v D.R.H, Unpub. LEXIS 3250 (NJ Super. Ct. Ch. Div. 2009). Although, as I noted back in Chapter 5, note 36 both of these cases came before *Obergefell v Hodges* (135 S. Ct. 2584, 2600-01) (2015).

[33] For a sense of where things stand in the United States: in 2017, the Uniform Law Commission, which provides states with "non-partisan, well-conceived and well-drafted legislation that brings clarity and stability to critical areas of state statutory law," introduced an updated version of the Uniform Parentage Act, which had last been updated in 2002. Among other things, the UPA 2017 seeks to ensure "the equal treatment of children born to same-sex couples. UPA (2002) was written in gendered terms, and its provisions presumed that couples consist of one man and one woman." With respect to the gamete donation, it introduces Article 9, which "does not require disclosure of the identity of a gamete donor, but does require gamete banks and fertility clinics to ask donors if they want to have their identifying information disclosed when the resulting child attains 18 years of age. It does require disclosure of non-identifying medical history of the gamete donor." National Conference of Commissioners on Uniform State Laws, "Uniform Parentage Act (2017)," 2017. https://www.uniformlaws.org/HigherLogic/System/DownloadDocumentFile. ashx?DocumentFileKey=e4a82c2a-f7cc-b33e-ed68-47ba88c36d92&forceDialog=0.

[34] Kirk Makin, "Two Mothers Should Be Allowed on Birth Document, Judge Says," *Globe and Mail*, June 7, 2006, https://www.theglobeandmail.com/news/national/two-mothers-should-be-allowed-on-birth-document-judge-says/article710237/.

The situation for gay parents that used a *known* donor, however, remained more complicated. Until 2017, the non-biological parent in a same-sex couple that used a known donor could not be automatically registered as a parent on their child's birth certificate. As a result, the non-biological parent needed to adopt their own child in order to be legally recognized as a parent. The burdens that this imposed on same-sex couples were brought to the fore by the experience of Jennifer Mathers McHenry, who experienced a difficult childbirth. As she recounts, "There was a moment where [my wife] Kirsti wasn't so sure either I was going to come home, and if I didn't, if she could bring our baby home, so that really drove home the degree to which the law puts families like ours in limbo."[35] Of course, the law imposed a burden on same-sex couples even absent such an extreme situation, since the non-biological parent needed to go through the process of adopting their child. And their parental status was not legally recognized until the adoption was completed. More generally, the law evinced a bionormative view about which families are "real" from the get-go and which deserve special scrutiny. As Alice MacLachlan and Amy Noseworthy put it:

> When families like [ours] are excluded from systems of birth registration and parental recognition, then parents just like us are told that we are not good enough and we do not count, and that our rights are somehow precarious, while our friends' and neighbours' rights are not. Children just like [ours] are told their families are secondary, and only second best.[36]

This all changed in 2017 when a group of parents—including MacLachlan and Noseworthy—brought a Charter challenge, which ultimately led to the passage of the All Families Are Equal Act. Among other things, the new law replaces the terms "mother" and "father" with "parent" and allows the birth parent to enter into a preconception parenting agreement with up to four people.[37]

---

[35] Allison Jones, "New Ontario Act Ensures Same-Sex Couples Won't Have to Adopt Own Kids," *Globe and Mail*, September 29, 2016, https://www.theglobeandmail.com/news/national/ontario-to-change-law-that-requires-same-sex-couples-to-adopt-own-kids/article32127031/.

[36] Alice MacLachlan and Amy Noseworthy, "By Ignoring Parental Rights, Ontario Puts Our Daughter's Welfare at Risk," *Globe and Mail*, June 2, 2016, https://www.theglobeandmail.com/opinion/by-ignoring-parental-rights-ontario-puts-our-daughters-welfare-at-risk/article30244298/.

[37] Allison Jones, "All Families Are Equal Act Passes: Same-Sex Parents in Ontario Won't Have to Adopt Own Kids," *HuffPost*, November 30, 2016, https://www.huffingtonpost.ca/2016/11/30/all-families-are-equal-act-bill-28-wynne_n_13326140.html. There are still significant obstacles in Ontario (at least) for intended parents that want to use a known donor. The process is considerably more costly (if you use a clinic) and requires multiple counselling sessions for both intended parents

Education. Anyone familiar with debates about abstinence-only sex education will be unsurprised to learn that a significant portion of sex education in the United States is explicitly geared toward presenting the bionormative family as *the* desired family form. Indeed, The Personal Responsibility and Work Opportunity Reconciliation Act of 1996 created funding for sex education that (among other things) "teaches abstinence from sexual activity outside marriage as the expected standard for all school age children" and "teaches that a mutually faithful monogamous relationship in the context of marriage is the expected standard of human sexual activity."[38] As Tanya McNeill remarks, "Curricula that promote abstinence—particularly abstinence until marriage—assume that full belonging as an adult and a citizen in the community, family, and nation requires heteronormative family relations."[39]

Perhaps more telling, however, are curricula that aimed for greater inclusion but still reinforced bionormativity. Consider two examples from recent history, one from Prince William County School District in Virginia and the other from California's 2003 *Health Framework for California Public Schools: Kindergarten through Grade Twelve:*

> Teachers will teach that, although it is desirable for a family to include both a mother and a father, due to circumstances beyond the control of a child, this does not always occur. As many children in a classroom will not have a traditional family, the teacher should reinforce that these children should not feel "less worthy" because their family does not resemble the family of other students.[40]

and the prospective donor. In general, the plan to use a known (rather than an open or anonymous) donor is greeted with skepticism by clinics. The presence of such obstacles is relevant for what I say below about whether intended parents should use a known donor (p. 213).

[38] The Personal Responsibility and Work Opportunity Reconciliation Act of 1996, Pub. L. No. 104–193, 110 STAT. 2105 (1996).

[39] McNeill puts the point even more strongly: "The juxtaposition of the description of two-parent heterosexual, married families with a discussion of 'non-traditional' families (and the use of the word 'however') implies that non-heteronormative families are not 'functional,' 'stable' or 'consistent' and that they are unlikely to offer the same level of 'love, support, and direction' as 'traditional' families can." Tanya McNeill, "Sex Education and the Promotion of Heteronormativity," *Sexualities* 16, no. 7 (2013): 832.

[40] Prince William County Public Schools, *Family Life Education Grade 8 Health: Curriculum Objectives For Use In Mapping Family Life Education Instruction* August 2009. This document no longer appears online. The most recent version of the Family Health curriculum has dropped this language. The first grade curriculum, for example, now says the following:

> "Students learn that although every family is different, all families are important for providing love, support, security, understanding, and care. Family structures include

A functional family unit is vital to the well-being of children. Children usually develop best when they live in a stable environment with their mother and father and receive from their parents consistent love, support, and direction. However, children from nontraditional families can also develop successfully. Given the variety of nontraditional families in contemporary society, it is important that children not reared in two-parent families be convinced that their situation can also be conducive to growth and development.[41]

Both documents clearly established the bionormative family as the model of proper family life. The Virginia document identified the bionormative family as "desirable." And while it acknowledged that children from nontraditional families should not be made to feel "less worthy," it implies that this should be done only because it is not the child's fault that they find themselves in a family situation that is less than ideal.

The California document identified the bionormative family as the one where children "usually" develop best. And while other family forms are also credited with being able to function well, the document expresses something close to surprise about this possibility ("However, children from nontraditional families can also develop successfully") and seems to suggest that conditions must be just right in order for it to actually come to pass ("it is important that children not reared in two-parent families be convinced that their situation can also be conducive to growth and development").[42] As McNeill notes, "According to these state policies, teachers in California

two-parent families; extended families—relatives other than the immediate family living in the home; single-parent families; adoptive families; foster families; families with stepparents; and blended families."

However, there are still vestiges of heteronormativity. In the fifth grade FLE curriculum, for example, "Students are introduced to the concept that babies originate from the uniting of the egg and the sperm through sexual intercourse." See Prince William County Public Schools, Family Life Education, Elementary School Objectives, https://www.pwcs.edu/academics___programs/science___family_life_education/family_life_education

[41] Curriculum Development and Supplemental Materials Commission, *Health Framework for California Public Schools Kindergarten Through Grade Twelve*, California Department of Education, Sacramento, 2003, 63. The 2019 guidelines are considerably improved on this front. They note that, "students learn that there are different family structures in our society and that all family structures are valid" and that "teachers should not assume a student lives in any particular family structure and should ask questions in a way that will easily include children from diverse family backgrounds ensuring sensitivity to family diversity and privacy." Curriculum Frameworks and Instructional Resources Division, *Health Framework for California Public Schools Kindergarten Through Grade Twelve*, California Department of Education, Sacramento, 2019.

[42] McNeill, "Sex Education and the Promotion of Heteronormativity," 833.

and in Prince William County must simultaneously teach their students that the heteropatriarchal family is most 'desirable' and manage (or discipline) the negative feelings that might emerge for students whose families look 'different.' "[43]

A little later she observes that these kinds of policies raise an "affective pedagogical problem" when students are asked to do assignments that involve identifying members of one's family. "What kind of reception," McNeill asks, "do we imagine that a student with lesbian mothers, gay fathers, or other non-normative family forms will receive within the classroom? What would it feel like to be five years old and identify your family as 'different'?"[44]

Individual behavior. We saw various examples back in chapter 5 of individual behavior that evinces bionormative prejudice: children who are confronted by other children with the question "Who is your father?"; a sign on Mother's Day that reads, "She birthed you! Buy her a beer!"; a song that celebrates genetic connectedness as the basis for what makes people family. In myriad ways big and small we tend to convey that family relatedness—what it means to be a mother or a father or a daughter or a son—is grounded in genetic relatedness or, more mythically, "blood." The problem here is not so much with any individual behavior viewed in isolation, but with the ubiquity of such behavior. Taken together, they serve to reinforce the idea that genetic (or more broadly biological) connectedness is the *bona fide* form of family connectedness.

Perhaps the clearest manifestation of this commitment at the level of individual behavior is the popularity of the "resemblance game" wherein people remark on just how similar people presumed to be genetically related are to each other. People routinely play the game with their own family ("You have your father's ears") and other people's family, including total strangers ("She is just a spitting image of you!"). As Haslanger puts it:

> What similarities are salient is largely a matter of context, and some socially significant similarities are allowed to eclipse others that may be more deeply important. I don't really see our physical similarities, but [Haslanger's adopted son] Isaac and I have other emotional and temperamental

---

[43] McNeill, "Sex Education and the Promotion of Heteronormativity," 836. Though as noted above, the curricular requirements have improved considerably in the intervening years.

[44] McNeill, "Sex Education and the Promotion of Heteronormativity," 835–36. Recall that this is precisely the kind of bionormativity we saw back in chapter 5 that confronted McLeod's adopted son when asked to do an assignment about how his mother and grandfather reacted to his birth.

similarities. This too can be easily eclipsed by our racial (and sex) difference. Social schemas tell us, among other things: Who are you allowed to
look like? Who are you allowed to *be* like?[45]

The problem is that the resemblance game tends to focus on one *kind* of
similarity, namely physical similarity that is (presumed to be) genetically
transmitted. These similarities are taken to mark parents and children as
"really" related, as "properly" belonging together. As a result, other kinds of
similarity—including those that are plausibly more meaningful than physical similarity, like "emotional and temperamental similarities"—are either
attributed to genetic relatedness[46] or downgraded as a less significant mark
of relatedness (if they are noticed at all).

I don't mean to suggest that any of this is conscious. Rather it manifests
when people behold a striking physical resemblance between a parent and
child and remark, "There's no doubt he's your son!" or "She's just a mini-
version of her mother!" Likewise, it manifests in the *lack* of remarks of this
sort[47] when there is a presumption that there is no genetic connection between parent and child. The message to people who cannot play the game in
the culturally appropriate way is clear: you (and your parents) are missing the
thing that really ties families together.

These are three illustrations from three domains—law, education, and individual behavior—of policies and practices that reinforce bionormativity.
These kinds of policies and practices (not to mention many others in other
domains) ought to be changed as part of any effort to prohibit anonymous
gamete donation, lest such efforts serve to reinforce the prejudice that non-
traditional families already face. One important consequence of this point
is that the question of whether anonymous gamete donation should be
allowed does not just affect members of the donor-conception community.
Instead, it affects all of us for the simple reason that the task of combating
bionormativity falls on all of our shoulders.

So here's where we are. I have argued throughout the book that intended parents should use an open donor. But the decision about whether
to use an open or anonymous donor—and so the option of choosing

---

[45] Sally Haslanger, "Family, Ancestry, and Self," in *Resisting Reality: Social Construction and Social Critique* (New York: Oxford University Press, 2012), 170.

[46] Recall the examples of genetic essentialism in chapter 4.

[47] As Haslanger recounts, "[A] female friend with two sons once commented that my son Isaac and I look alike. I was surprised since no one had ever mentioned this before." Haslanger, "Family, Ancestry, and Self," 170.

wrongly—properly belongs with intended parents, at least until efforts to prohibit anonymous gamete donation are accompanied by real work to substantially disrupt the bionormative schema.

4. Using a known donor

I want to conclude the book by turning to a question I raised way back in chapter 1: Do my arguments for using an open donor imply that intended parents should choose a *known* donor, i.e. a donor whose identity will be known to the child from a young age?

I don't propose to offer anything like an exhaustive answer to this question. Part of the reason is that such an answer would depend on data we just don't have concerning the outcomes—for children, but also for parents—of using a known donor versus an open donor. Learning that things worked considerably better one way or the other (for children or parents or both) could easily settle the matter. Absent such data, any answer to our question must be tentative. Moreover, the practical difficulties of identifying and, in effect, negotiating with a potential known donor prevent any argument I have made from establishing that, in general, intended parents should use a known donor. Even so, I want to finish by pointing to two reasons my argument for using an open donor provisionally suggests that intended parents should, if possible, seriously consider choosing a known donor.

First, people (donor-conceived and non-donor-conceived alike) typically start asking the identity questions I talked about in chapter 4 before the age of 18. Indeed, a hallmark of teenage years is that you start to form a self-conception, to tell a story (to yourself and others) about your place in the world, about who you are. In other words, the significant interest that many donor-conceived people develop will come online before the age of 18. That gives parents at least some reason to put the child in a position to satisfy the interest before 18.

Other considerations could point in the other direction. Perhaps we'll learn, over time, that giving donor-conceived people access to genetic knowledge prior to 18 is a bad idea. Perhaps it interferes with family functioning in a way that is especially deleterious to the well-being of the child or parents. Or perhaps, given our bionormative world, providing access to genetic knowledge prior to 18 serves to reinforce biogenetic prejudice by effectively saying, "Here is important information you *must* have," and so perhaps it should be resisted for that reason. Maybe it is better to keep the child insulated from genetic knowledge for 18 years in an effort to get them to form—or at least appreciate the possibility of forming—an identity that does not depend on having genetic knowledge.

I think there are two good reasons to be skeptical of these ideas. First, it is not realistically possible, within the bounds of acceptable parenting, to keep questions about genetic knowledge off a donor-conceived child's radar until they are 18. Second, giving a child access to genetic knowledge from an early age is, I suggest, the *most* effective way of rendering the knowledge relatively irrelevant to the child. Let's take each reason in turn.

The first point is, I hope, obvious by now. As I argued way back in chapter 2, parents of donor-conceived children should disclose to their child they are donor-conceived basically as soon as the child is capable of understanding.[48] Keeping a child's donor-conceived status secret is wrong not only because it is likely to be harmful to the child—given the impact of likely discovery later in life—but also because it involves an unacceptable form of parental deception about the nature of their relationship with their child. There is no morally acceptable way of insulating a donor-conceived child from questions about their genetic lineage until they are 18. Given that disclosure is morally required, the only real choice is between having and not having access to genetic knowledge at the time of disclosure.

What about the concern that providing genetic knowledge early on will only serve to reinforce bionormativity? This brings us to my second reason for thinking that parents should make genetic information available from an early age: if the goal is to *not* give genetic knowledge an aura of significance that it should not have, then providing genetic knowledge early is more effective than the alternative. This is an empirical conjecture. But it is based on an undeniable feature of human psychology: making something forbidden is a very effective way to make it attractive (see: the Garden of Eden). Making genetic information unavailable effectively presents a donor-conceived child with a black box that reads: "Herein lies something serious, something you cannot handle right now." That approach seems perfectly designed to pique, rather than abate, an interest in having genetic knowledge. Indeed, in the absence of genetic knowledge, donor-conceived people often fantasize about

---

[48] And that is an ongoing process: very early explanations will be very different than later explanations, and explanations will need to be offered again and again before there is genuine uptake.

their donor—about what he is like, about what it would be like to meet him.[49] It is as though their parents have hung a picture in their room, but covered it with a sign that reads, "Not to be viewed until older." Who could stop thinking about what is behind the sign? Indeed, Hertz and Nelson report that donor-conceived children "who want to solve the mystery of who the donor is . . . have no choice but to complete the process of constructing the donor with their own imagination."[50]

Contrast this approach, which we might call the *black-box* strategy, with what we might call the *fish-in-water* strategy, where a donor-conceived person knows that she is donor-conceived and has known who the donor is for as long as she can remember. It is simply a feature of her life, one that has always been with her. No part of her psychic economy will be devoted to wondering—indeed, fantasizing—about it. As we saw in chapter 2, secrets sometimes hide something significant. But oftentimes, secrecy *creates* significance.

Now, I've argued that people's interest in genetic knowledge is not groundless. The interest can be a genuine site of identity determination. So I do not claim that the black-box approach creates the significance of genetic knowledge. But it is very plausible that it *inflates* it in the mind of the donor-conceived person. The fish-in-water strategy prevents that from happening. If the fish-in-water strategy were the norm, then perhaps donor-conceived people would not—as a rule—develop a significant interest (or as significant an interest) in genetic knowledge.

This leads to an ironic conclusion: if intended parents want to prevent their donor-conceived child from developing an interest in genetic knowledge that outstrips its genuine significance (and which is, perhaps, an expression of, and further entrenches, bionormative prejudice), then they should give the child access to that knowledge as early as possible. Other strategies will exacerbate, not mitigate, the problem.

Even if genetic information is made available at an early age, a lot will depend on *how* it is made available. If it is presented as something hugely significant ("Come child. We must now have a serious discussion about something very important."), then it is more likely to be taken up that way by the child.

---

[49] Amanda J. Turner and Adrian Coyle, "What Does It Mean to Be a Donor Offspring? The Identity Experiences of Adults Conceived by Donor Insemination and the Implications for Counselling and Therapy," *Human Reproduction* 15, no. 9 (2000): 2046.

[50] Rosanna Hertz and Margaret K. Nelson, *Random Families: Genetic Strangers, Sperm Donor Siblings, and the Creation of New Kin* (New York: Oxford University Press, 2018), 46.

But it needn't be done like that. Rather, it can be presented as a simple matter of fact, one that isn't imbued (in advance) with tremendous significance either by its glaring absence or by being accorded a tremendous weight in the telling.

Everyone has a story about how they came to be, woven from the hundreds, the thousands (tens of thousands!) of strands that came together to produce *them*. Which strands jump out and which fade into the background, which are imbued with profound significance and which are filler, which arouse curiosity and which pass as matters of indifference is not a *fait accompli*. We—as children, as parents, as extended family, as friends—are the weavers. We choose the threads that make the pattern. The thread of donor conception *should* be in the weave. The task is to find a place for it in the pattern that gives it its due, but no more.

Afterword

You are at the end of a book devoted to the ethics of conceiving children with donated gametes. Perhaps you, like many others I've discussed some of these ideas with over the past five years, are wondering: What got me interested in this topic?

I gave one answer in the first chapter. The questions at the heart of this book—*What is the value of genetic ties? To what extent must parents help their child pursue their (the child's) interests? What is parental responsibility and how do you get it?*—matter for everyone, including me. Everyone has a family of one kind or another. And everyone has at least a nascent theory of families and parenthood that probably plays a significant role in how they live their lives. Thinking about the ethics of gamete donation is a very productive way of thinking about relationships that are central to people's lives, including mine.

All that is absolutely true. But there is more to say. To get at that "more," let me describe a photograph.[1] I am in it, along with my wife and two children, Eleanor and Aubin. To our left is my mother, Lucille. To our right is my sister Colette. And to Colette's right is a woman named Joane. Joane is Colette's birthmother. My other two sisters—Rachelle and Dianne—are not in the picture. But we can imagine that they are. And that next to them are *their* birthmothers. My birthmother is also in the picture, but I've already mentioned her—it's Lucille.

I am the biological child of my social mother. My sisters, on the other hand, were all adopted. I've known that for as long as I can remember and,

---

[1] It's a real photograph, although I've changed some of the details.

as far as I know, so have they. I grew up in a family where questions about relatedness, the significance of genetic ties, and what makes a family *a family* were never far from the surface. Sometimes, they would burst into the open, such as when, at age 5, I told my youngest sister I wish she had never been adopted or when a friend of mine in the sixth grade took to calling my sisters "phonies."

My parents were unequivocal in their view that we are all their children in the fullest sense of the term. Rachelle and Colette would be the first to tell you that being adopted has played no small part in their lives. For Dianne, "Being adopted has played a relatively small part in my life. It's simply another part of life. It's like having brown eyes—I have them. I am adopted. I think people who aren't adopted think it's a much bigger deal than it often is (for the adoptee)." I like that one of the central points in my book—namely, that an interest in one's genetic origins is rationally optional—is reflected in my own family.

So, how could I not be interested in the questions at the heart of this book? They have been present for me for as long as I can remember. But even that is not the full story. Let's return to the photograph. Standing next to my mother is my very close friend Alice and next to her is her wife, Amy. Standing in front of them are their two daughters, Emmylou and Martha. Their daughters are my genetic offspring.

When Alice and Amy got married, they mentioned to my wife and me that they were planning to conceive with a donor and that they would like to use a known donor. Not long after that—and in consultation with my spouse—I offered to be their donor. It was not a hard decision for us. We did not struggle with infertility. We already had a child, who we jokingly referred to as the "floor model," whenever the topic of gamete donation came up with Alice and Amy. We were very happy to help two people we love—and who love each other—form a family. Indeed, my wife and I barely spent any time thinking about it, which is not to say that we didn't take it seriously. It just struck us as something we would like to do.

The ideas for this book only arose after the fact as I started to think more deeply about what it means to be a gamete donor and as I read what other people think about gamete donation. As you know by now, the conclusion I argue for in the book is that if you're going to conceive children with donated gametes, the donor's identity should be known—or at least accessible—to the donor-conceived child. And hey! That means the decision I (and my wife and Alice and Amy) made was the right one! Phew!

You can now see why I started this afterword with the quote from Nietzsche. This book is not great philosophy. But it is undeniably a kind of memoir. In my more cynical moments, I wonder whether the arguments I've made over hundreds of pages are nothing more than a post-hoc rationalization for a decision I made without much reflection. But I hope that's not the case. Instead, I'm inclined to believe that a person's values can be present in, and live through, them without ever being articulated, let alone formulated into a sustained argument that takes up a book. This is not to say that everything in the preceding pages was already present, however implicitly, in my decision to be a donor. There are certainly parts of the book that I had no antecedent views about and others where I changed my mind partway through writing. But the core thought—that donors should be known to donor-conceived children—was already present, I think, in my decision to become a donor in the way, and for the people, that I did.

It mattered for all of us that our families are close friends, that Emmylou and Martha's origins will never be a secret, that we are in touch a lot, and that we all get together regularly (albeit infrequently). Most importantly, we are all open to, and open-minded about, the complexities that might be coming down the road as not just Emmylou and Martha, but also my children, grow up and forge their own understanding of how our families are related (in more than one sense of the term). There is richness in this complexity, the possibility for exploring sources of meaning or pursuing paths for identity-determination that come from having what Alice calls an "abundant family configuration."[2]

So, that is the full story of how I became interested in the topic. I've shared it as an afterword and not a foreword because I hope the arguments I've made in the preceding pages stand on their own, neither gaining nor losing strength in the reader's mind because they know I am a donor. But maybe, now that you know, the arguments in the preceding pages will take on a different hue. Best turn back to the first page and start again.

[2] Alice MacLachlan, "Conceiving Differently within the Ethics of Assisted Reproduction," *APA Newsletter on LGBTQ Issues in Philosophy* 19, no. 1 (2019): 14.

Bibliography

Adoption Network. "US Adoption Statistics." Accessed August 3, 2020. https://adoptionnetwork.com/adoption-statistics.

Anonymous Us. "I Have Never Met My Donor 'Father' and I Have No Desire to Do So." October 31, 2011. https://anonymousus.org/i-have-never-met-my-donor-father-and-i-have-no-desire-to-do-so/.

A.G.R. v D.R.H, Unpub. LEXIS 3250 (NJ Super. Ct. Ch. Div. 2009).

Ahuja, Kamal K. "Is the UK Sperm Donor Shortage a Myth?" *BioNews*, May 2015. https://www.bionews.org.uk/page_95041.

Almeling, Rene. "Opinion: The Unregulated Sperm Industry." *New York Times*, November 30, 2013. https://www.nytimes.com/2013/12/01/opinion/sunday/the-unregulated-sperm-industry.html.

Almeling, Rene. *Sex Cells: The Medical Market for Eggs and Sperm*. Berkeley: University of California Press, 2011.

Appell, Annette. "The Endurance of Biological Connection: Heteronormativity, Same-Sex Parenting and the Lessons of Adoption." *BYU Journal of Public Law* 22, no. 2 (2008): 289–326.

Appleby, John B., Lucy Blake, and Tabitha Freeman. "Is Disclosure in the Best Interests of Children Conceived by Donation?," edited by M. Richards, G. Pennings, & J. Appleby, *Reproductive Donation: Practice, Policy and Bioethics*, 231–249. Cambridge: Cambridge University Press, 2012.

Appleby, John B., and Anja Karnein. "On the Moral Importance of Genetic Ties in Families." In *Relatedness in Assisted Reproduction: Families, Origins and Identities*, edited by T. Freeman, F. Ebtehaj, S. Graham, and M. Richards, 79–96. Cambridge: Cambridge University Press, 2014.

Archard, David. "The Obligations and Responsibilities of Parenthood." In *Procreation and Parenthood: The Ethics of Bearing and Rearing Children*, edited by David Archard and David Benatar. 103–127. New York: Oxford University Press, 2010.

Baden, Amanda L., Doug Shadel, Ron Morgan, Ebony E. White, Elliotte S. Harrington, Nicole Christian, and Todd A. Bates. "Delaying Adoption Disclosure: A Survey of Late Discovery Adoptees." *Journal of Family Issues*, 1154–1180. May 14, 2019.

Baker, Kate. Twitter post. November 18th, 2020, 2.20pm. https://twitter.com/BakeKater/status/1329157443356528641

Baldwin, James. *The Fire Next Time*. New York: Knopf Doubleday, 2013.

Bartky, Sandra Lee. *Femininity and Domination: Studies in the Phenomenology of Oppression*. New York: Routledge, 2015.

Bayne, Tim. "Gamete Donation and Parental Responsibility." *Journal of Applied Philosophy* 20, no. 1 (2003): 77–87.

Becker, Gay, Anneliese Butler, and Robert D. Nachtigall. "Resemblance Talk: A Challenge for Parents Whose Children Were Conceived with Donor Gametes in the US." *Social Science & Medicine* 61, no. 6 (2005): 1300–1309.

Beeson, Diane R., Patricia K. Jennings, and Wendy Kramer. "Offspring Searching for Their Sperm Donors: How Family Type Shapes the Process." *Human Reproduction* 26, no. 9 (2011): 2415–24.

Benatar, David. *Better Never to Have Been: The Harm of Coming into Existence.* New York: Oxford University Press, 2008.

Benatar, David. "The Unbearable Lightness of Bringing into Being." *Journal of Applied Philosophy* 16, no. 2 (1999): 173–80.

Bengtson, Vern L., Susan Harris, and Norella M. Putney. *Families and Faith: How Religion Is Passed Down across Generations.* New York: Oxford University Press, 2017.

Benson, Paul. "Autonomy and Oppressive Socialization." *Social Theory and Practice* 17, no. 3 (1991): 385–408.

Benward, J., J. R. Guichon, I. Mitchell, and M. Giroux. "Identity Development in the Donor-Conceived Child." In *The Right to Know One's Origins: Assisted Human Reproduction and the Best Interests of Children*, edited by Juliet Ruth Guichon, Ian Mitchell, and Michelle Giroux, 166–91. Brussels: ASP, 2012.

Block, Ned. "Race, Genes, and IQ." *Boston Review*, May 5, 2017. http://bostonreview.net/science-nature-race/ned-block-race-genes-and-iq.

Bloom, P. Artificial insemination (donor).The Eugenics Review, 48, 1957, 205–207.

Botterell, Andrew. "Why Gametes Are Not Like Enriched Uranium." *Bioethics* 30, no. 9 (2016): 741–50.

Bowles, Nellie. "The Sperm Kings Have a Problem: Too Much Demand." *New York Times*, January 8, 2021. https://www.nytimes.com/2021/01/08/business/sperm-donors-facebook-groups.html.

Brake, Elizabeth. "Willing Parents: A Voluntarist Account of Parental Role Obligations." In *Procreation and Parenthood: The Ethics of Bearing and Rearing Children*, edited by David Archard and David Benatar, 151–177. New York: Oxford University Press, 2010.

Brandt, Reuven. "The Transfer and Delegation of Responsibilities for Genetic Offspring in Gamete Provision." *Journal of Applied Philosophy* 34, no. 5 (2017): 665–78.

Brennan, Samantha. "The Goods of Childhood, Children's Rights, and the Role of Parents as Advocates and Interpreters." In *Family-Making: Contemporary Ethical Challenges*, edited by F. Baylis and C. McLeod, 29–48. n.d. New York: Oxford University Press.

Briggs, Laura. *Somebody's Children: The Politics of Transracial and Transnational Adoption.* Durham, NC: Duke University Press, 2012.

Brighouse, Harry, and Adam Swift. *Family Values: The Ethics of Parent-Child Relationships.* Princeton, NJ: Princeton University Press, 2014.

Buller, David J. "Evolutionary Psychology: The Emperor's New Paradigm." *Trends in Cognitive Sciences* 9, no. 6 (June 2005): 277–83.

Cahn, Naomi R. *The New Kinship: Constructing Donor-Conceived Families.* New York: NYU Press, 2013.

California Cryobank. "Donor Types." Accessed January 12, 2021. https://www.cryobank.com/how-it-works/donor-types/.

CBC News. "Fertility Doctor Implanted Own Sperm in Clients 11 Times, Lawsuit Alleges." April 5, 2018. https://www.cbc.ca/news/canada/ottawa/fertility-doctor-own-sperm-11-times-1.4606814.CBS Chicago. "Man Conceived at Des Plaines Oasis Stages One-Man Protest of Closure." March 14, 2014. https://chicago.cbslocal.com/2014/03/14/man-conceived-at-des-plaines-oasis-stages-one-man-protest-of-closure/.

Cha, Ariana Eunjung. "Her 44 Siblings Were Conceived with One Donor's Sperm: Here's How It Was Possible." *Washington Post*, September 12, 2018. https://www.washingtonpost.com/graphics/2018/health/44-donor-siblings-and-counting/.

Chideya, Farai. "Excuse Me, May I Raise Your Child?" *Medium*, July 8, 2019. https://zora.medium.com/excuse-me-may-i-raise-your-child-45afc26f088d.

"Cinderella Effect." Wikipedia, August 8, 2020. https://en.wikipedia.org/w/index.php?title=Cinderella_effect&oldid=971884222.

Clark, Katrina. "Who's Your Daddy?" *Washington Post*, December 17, 2006. https://www.washingtonpost.com/archive/opinions/2006/12/17/whos-your-daddy/856d8f09-d17c-4a0c-be1b-5435190b084c/.

Clayton, Matthew. "Anti-Perfectionist Childrearing." In *The Nature of Children's Well-Being*, edited by Alexander Bagattini and Colin Macleod, 123–40. New York: Springer, 2015.

Clayton, Matthew. *Justice and Legitimacy in Upbringing*. New York: Oxford University Press, 2006.

CoParents. "Artificial Insemination: The Turkey Baster Method." Accessed August 2, 2020. https://www.coparents.com/blog/the-turkey-baster-method-what-is-it-and-how-to-perform-it/.

Corvino, John. "My Daddy's Name Is 'Donor.'" Blog. June 4, 2010. https://www.johncorvino.com/2010/06/04/my-daddys-name-is-donor/.

Crawshaw, Marilyn, Damian Adams, Sonia Allan, Eric Blyth, Kate Bourne, Claudia Brügge, Anne Chien, et al. "Disclosure and Donor-Conceived Children." *Human Reproduction* 32, no. 7 (July 1, 2017): 1535–36.

Curriculum Development and Supplemental Materials Commission, *Health Framework for California Public Schools Kindergarten Through Grade Twelve*, California Department of Education, Sacramento, 2003.

Curriculum Frameworks and Instructional Resources Division, **Health Framework for California Public Schools Kindergarten Through Grade Twelve**, , California Department of Education, Sacramento, 2019.

Dickinson, Amy. "Perspective: Ask Amy: DNA Testing Reveals Shocking Results." *Washington Post*, February 13, 2018. https://www.washingtonpost.com/lifestyle/style/ask-amy-dna-testing-reveals-shocking-results/2018/02/13/54097586-076a-11e8-b48c-b07fea957bd5_story.html.

Doe v. Doe, 710 A.2d 1297 (Conn. 1998).

Dominus, Susan. "The Mixed-Up Brothers of Bogotá." *New York Times*, July 9, 2015. https://www.nytimes.com/2015/07/12/magazine/the-mixed-up-brothers-of-bogota.html.

Dominus, Susan. "Sperm Donors Can't Stay Secret Anymore: Here's What That Means." *New York Times*, June 26, 2019. https://www.nytimes.com/2019/06/26/magazine/sperm-donor-questions.html.

Dub, Richard. "Delusions, Acceptances, and Cognitive Feelings." *Philosophy and Phenomenological Research* 94, no. 1 (2017): 27–60.

Du Bois, William Edward Burghardt. *The Souls of Black Folk*. New York: Oxford University Press, 2008.

Ebels-Duggan, Kyla. "Against Beneficence: A Normative Account of Love." *Ethics* 119, no. 1 (2008): 142–70.

Ehrensaft, Diane. *Mommies, Daddies, Donors, Surrogates: Answering Tough Questions and Building Strong Families*. New York: Guilford Press, 2005.

Ekerhovd, Erling, and Anders Faurskov. "Swedish Sperm Donors Are Driven by Altruism, but Shortage of Sperm Donors Leads to Reproductive Travelling." *Upsala Journal of Medical Sciences* 113, no. 3 (2008): 305–14.

Erlich, Yaniv, Tal Shor, Itsik Pe'er, and Shai Carmi. "Identity Inference of Genomic Data Using Long-Range Familial Searches." *Science* 362, no. 6415 (November 9, 2018): 690–94.

Eyal, Nir, Samia A. Hurst, Christopher J. L. Murray, S. Andrew Schroeder, and Daniel Wikler. *Measuring the Global Burden of Disease: Philosophical Dimensions.* New York: Oxford University Press, 2020.

Feinberg, Joel. "The Child's Right to an Open Future." In *Justice, Politics, and the Family,* edited by Daniel Engster and Tamara Metz, 145–60. New York: Routledge, 2015.

Fessler, Ann. *The Girls Who Went Away: The Hidden History of Women Who Surrendered Children for Adoption in the Decades before Roe v. Wade.* New York: Penguin, 2007.

Frame, Thomas R. *Children on Demand: The Ethics of Defying Nature.* Sydney: UNSW Press, 2008.

Freeman, Tabitha, John B. Appleby, and Vasanti Jadva. "Identifiable Donors and Siblings." In *Reproductive Donation,* edited by Martin Richards, Guido Pennings, and John Appleby, 250–69. Cambridge: Cambridge University Press, 2012.

Freeman, Tabitha, Vasanti Jadva, Wendy Kramer, and Susan Golombok. "Gamete Donation: Parents' Experiences of Searching for Their Child's Donor Siblings and Donor." *Human Reproduction* 24, no. 3 (2009): 505–16.

Freeman, Tabitha, Sophie Zadeh, Venessa Smith, and Susan Golombok. "Disclosure of Sperm Donation: A Comparison between Solo Mother and Two-Parent Families with Identifiable Donors." *Reproductive Biomedicine Online* 33, no. 5 (2016): 592–600.

Fricker, Miranda. *Epistemic Injustice: Power and the Ethics of Knowing.* New York: Oxford University Press, 2007.

Frith, Lucy. "Beneath the Rhetoric: The Role of Rights in the Practice of Non-Anonymous Gamete Donation." *Bioethics* 15, nos. 5–6 (2001): 473–84.

Frith, Lucy. "Gamete Donation and Anonymity: The Ethical and Legal Debate." *Human Reproduction* 16, no. 5 (2001): 818–24.

Frith, Lucy, Eric Blyth, Marilyn Crawshaw, and Olga van den Akker. "Secrets and Disclosure in Donor Conception." *Sociology of Health & Illness* 40, no. 1 (2018): 188–203.

Frye, Marilyn. *The Politics of Reality: Essays in Feminist Theory.* Berkeley, CA: Crossing Press, 1983.

Fuscaldo, Giuliana. "Genetic Ties: Are They Morally Binding?" *Bioethics* 20, no. 2 (2006): 64–76.

Gheaus, Anca. "Biological Parenthood: Gestational, Not Genetic." *Australasian Journal of Philosophy* 96, no. 2 (April 3, 2018): 225–40.

Godman, Kate M., Katherine Sanders, Michael Rosenberg, and Peter Burton. "Potential Sperm Donors', Recipients' and Their Partners' Opinions towards the Release of Identifying Information in Western Australia." *Human Reproduction* 21, no. 11 (2006): 3022–26.

Gollancz, David. "Time to Stop Lying." *Guardian,* August 2, 2007. https://www.theguardian.com/society/2007/aug/02/childrensservices.humanrights.

Golombok, Susan. "Disclosure and Donor-Conceived Children." *Human Reproduction* 32, no. 7 (2017): 1532–1536.

Golombok, Susan. *Modern Families: Parents and Children in New Family Forms.* Cambridge: Cambridge University Press, 2015.

Golombok, Susan, Laura Mellish, Sarah Jennings, Polly Casey, Fiona Tasker, and Michael E. Lamb. "Adoptive Gay Father Families: Parent-Child Relationships and Children's Psychological Adjustment." *Child Development* 85, no. 2 (2014): 456–68.

Gottlieb, Claes, Othon Lalos, and Frank Lindblad. "Disclosure of Donor Insemination to the Child: The Impact of Swedish Legislation on Couples' Attitudes." *Human Reproduction* 15, no. 9 (2000): 2052–56.

Greenfeld, Dorothy A., and Susan Caruso Klock. "Disclosure Decisions among Known and Anonymous Oocyte Donation Recipients." *Fertility and Sterility* 81, no. 6 (2004): 1565–71.

Groll, Daniel. "Four Models of Family Interests." *Pediatrics* 134, Supplement 2 (2014): S81–S86.

Gudipati, Madhavi, Kim Pearce, Alka Prakash, Gillian Redhead, Victoria Hemingway, Kevin McEleny, and Jane Stewart. "The Sperm Donor Programme over 11 Years at Newcastle Fertility Centre." *Human Fertility* 16, no. 4 (2013): 258–65.

Guichon, Juliet Ruth, Ian Mitchell, and Michelle Giroux, eds. *The Right to Know One's Origins: Assisted Human Reproduction and the Best Interests of Children.* Brussels: ASP, 2012.

Hacking, Ian. *The social construction of what?* Cambridge, MA: Harvard University Press, 1999.

Hall, Ned. "Causal Contribution." In *Measuring the Global Burden of Disease: Philosophical Dimensions,* edited by Nir Eyal, Samia A. Hurst, Christopher J. L. Murray, S. Andrew Schroeder, and Daniel Wikler, 204–226. New York: Oxford University Press, 2020.

Hanna, Jason. "Causal Parenthood and the Ethics of Gamete Donation." *Bioethics* 33, no. 2 (2019): 267–73.

Hardwig, John. "What about the Family?" *Hastings Center Report* 20, no. 2 (1990): 5–10.

Harris, R., and L. Shanner. "Seeking Answers in the Ether: Longing to Know One's Origins Is Evident from Donor Conception Websites." In *The Right to Know One's Origins: Assisted Human Reproduction and the Best Interests of Children,* edited by Juliet Ruth Guichon, Ian Mitchell, and Michelle Giroux, 57–72. Brussels: ASP, 2012.

Haslanger, Sally. "Family, Ancestry, and Self." In *Resisting Reality: Social Construction and Social Critique,* 158–182. New York: Oxford University Press, 2012.

Hays, Sharon. *The Cultural Contradictions of Motherhood.* New Haven, CT: Yale University Press, 1996.

"Heritability," Wikipedia, December 2, 2020, https://en.wikipedia.org/w/index.php?title =Heritability&oldid=991870300.

Hertz, Rosanna, and Margaret K. Nelson. *Random Families: Genetic Strangers, Sperm Donor Siblings, and the Creation of New Kin.* New York: Oxford University Press, 2018.

"How to Order Donor Sperm." https://dk.cryosinternational.com/how-to/how-to-order-donor-sperm. Accessed February 2020.

Ishiguro, Kazuo. *Never Let Me Go.* London, England: Faber & Faber. 2010.

Jadva, Vasanti, Tabitha Freeman, Wendy Kramer, and Susan Golombok. "The Experiences of Adolescents and Adults Conceived by Sperm Donation: Comparisons by Age of Disclosure and Family Type." *Human Reproduction* 24, no. 8 (2009): 1909–19.

Jadva, Vasanti, Tabitha Freeman, Wendy Kramer, and Susan Golombok. "Experiences of Offspring Searching for and Contacting Their Donor Siblings and Donor." *Reproductive Biomedicine Online* 20, no. 4 (2010): 523–32.

Janssens, P. M. W., A. H. M. Simons, R. J. Van Kooij, E. Blokzijl, and G. A. J. Dunselman. "A New Dutch Law Regulating Provision of Identifying Information of Donors to Offspring: Background, Content and Impact." *Human Reproduction* 21, no. 4 (2006): 852–56.

Jones, Allison. "All Families Are Equal Act Passes: Same-Sex Parents in Ontario Won't Have to Adopt Own Kids." *HuffPost*, November 30, 2016. https://www.huffingtonpost.ca/2016/11/30/all-families-are-equal-act-bill-28-wynne_n_13326140.html.

Jones, Allison. "New Ontario Act Ensures Same-Sex Couples Won't Have to Adopt Own Kids." *Globe and Mail*, September 29, 2016. https://www.theglobeandmail.com/news/national/ontario-to-change-law-that-requires-same-sex-couples-to-adopt-own-kids/article32127031/.

Keller, Evelyn Fox. *The Mirage of a Space between Nature and Nurture*. Durham, NC: Duke University Press, 2010.

Klock, Susan C., and Donald Maier. "Psychological Factors Related to Donor Insemination." *Fertility and Sterility* 56, no. 3 (September 1, 1991): 489–95.

Kramer, Wendy, and Eric Blyth. " 'My Daddy's Name Is Donor': Read with Caution!" *BioNews*, July 9, 2010. https://www.bionews.org.uk/page_92455.

Lalos, Ann, Claes Gottlieb, and Othon Lalos. "Legislated Right for Donor-Insemination Children to Know Their Genetic Origin: A Study of Parental Thinking." *Human Reproduction* 22, no. 6 (2007): 1759–68.

Legal Aid Ontario. "Cy and Ruby's Law: Parental Recognition for Female Same-Sex Partners in Ontario." October 16, 2019. https://www.legalaid.on.ca/2019/10/16/cy-and-rubys-law-parental-recognition-for-female-same-sex-partners-in-ontario/.

Learn Genetics. "Observable Human Characteristics." Accessed March, 2019. https://learn.genetics.utah.edu/content/basics/observable/

Leighton, Kimberly. "Addressing the Harms of Not Knowing One's Heredity: Lessons from Genealogical Bewilderment." *Adoption & Culture* 3 (2012): 63–107.

Levy, Neil. "Forced to Be Free? Increasing Patient Autonomy by Constraining It." *Journal of Medical Ethics* 40, no. 5 (2014): 293–300.

Levy, Niel and Lotz, Mianna. "Reproductive Cloning and a (kind of) Genetic Fallacy." *Bioethics*, 19, no. 3 (2005): 232–250.

Lillehammer, Hallvard. "Who Cares Where You Come from? Cultivating Virtues of Indifference." In *Relatedness in Assisted Reproduction: Families, Origins and Identities*, edited by T. Freeman, F. Ebtehaj, S. Graham, and M. Richards, 97–112. Cambridge: Cambridge University Press, 2014.

Lindblad, F., C. Gottlieb, and O. Lalos. "To Tell or Not to Tell: What Parents Think about Telling Their Children That They Were Born Following Donor Insemination." *Journal of Psychosomatic Obstetrics & Gynecology* 21, no. 4 (2000): 193–203.

Livingston, Gretchen. "Fewer Than Half of US Kids Live in 'Traditional' Family." Pew Research Center (blog), December 22, 2014. https://www.pewresearch.org/fact-tank/2014/12/22/less-than-half-of-u-s-kids-today-live-in-a-traditional-family/.

Lugones, Maria C., and Elizabeth V. Spelman. "Have We Got a Theory for You! Feminist Theory, Cultural Imperialism and the Demand for 'the Woman's Voice.'" In *Women's Studies International Forum*, 6:573–81. Elsevier, 1983.

MacDougall, Kirstin, Gay Becker, Joanna E. Scheib, and Robert D. Nachtigall. "Strategies for Disclosure: How Parents Approach Telling Their Children That They Were Conceived with Donor Gametes." *Fertility and Sterility* 87, no. 3 (2007): 524–33.

MacLachlan, Alice. "Conceiving Differently within the Ethics of Assisted Reproduction." *APA Newsletter on LGBTQ Issues in Philosophy* 19, no. 1 (2019): 21.

MacLachlan, Alice, and Amy Noseworthy. "By Ignoring Parental Rights, Ontario Puts Our Daughter's Welfare at Risk." *Globe and Mail*, June 2, 2016. https://www.theglobeandmail.com/opinion/by-ignoring-parental-rights-ontario-puts-our-daughters-welfare-at-risk/article30244298/.

MacLeod, Colin. "Parental Responsibilities in an Unjust World." In *Procreation and Parenthood: The Ethics of Bearing and Rearing Children*, edited by David Archard and David Benatar, 128–150. New York: Oxford University Press, 2010.

Makin, Kirk. "Two Mothers Should Be Allowed on Birth Document, Judge Says." *Globe and Mail*, June 7, 2006. https://www.theglobeandmail.com/news/national/two-mothers-should-be-allowed-on-birth-document-judge-says/article710237/.

Marquardt, Elizabeth, Norval D. Glenn, and Karen Clark. *My Daddy's Name Is Donor: A New Study of Young Adults Conceived through Sperm Donation*. New York: Institute for American Values, 2010.

Martin, Walter. *Hey Sister* (New York: Family Jukebox, 2014).

McGee, Glenn, Sarah-Vaughan Brakman, and Andrea D. Gurmankin. "Gamete Donation and Anonymity: Disclosure to Children Conceived with Donor Gametes Should Not Be Optional." *Human Reproduction* 16, no. 10 (2001): 2033–36.

McNeill, Tanya. "Sex Education and the Promotion of Heteronormativity." *Sexualities* 16, no. 7 (2013): 826–46.

McTernan, Emily. "Should Fertility Treatment Be State Funded?" *Journal of Applied Philosophy* 32, no. 3 (2015): 227–40. https://doi.org/10.1111/japp.12091.

Medicine, Ethics Committee of the American Society for Reproductive. "Informing Offspring of Their Conception by Gamete Donation." *Fertility and Sterility* 81, no. 3 (2004): 527–31.

Melo-Martín, Inmaculada De. "The Ethics of Anonymous Gamete Donation: Is There a Right to Know One's Genetic Origins?" *Hastings Center Report* 44, no. 2 (2014): 28–35.

Mill, John Stuart. *"On Liberty" and Other Writings*. Cambridge Texts in the History of Political Thought. Cambridge: Cambridge University Press, 1989.

Mill, John Stuart. *Utilitarianism: And the 1868 Speech on Capital Punishment*. Hackett Classics. Indianapolis, IN: Hackett, 2002.

Mills, Claudia. "The Child's Right to an Open Future?" *Journal of Social Philosophy* 34, no. 4 (2003): 499–509.

Millum, Joseph. "How Do We Acquire Parental Responsibilities?" *Social Theory and Practice* 34, no. 1 (2008): 71.

Moller, Dan. "Wealth, Disability, and Happiness." *Philosophy & Public Affairs* no. 2 (2011): 177–206.

Mroz, Jacqueline. "A Mother Learns the Identity of Her Child's Grandmother: A Sperm Bank Threatens to Sue." *New York Times*, February 16, 2019. https://www.nytimes.com/2019/02/16/health/sperm-donation-dna-testing.html.

Mroz, Jacqueline. "Their Mothers Chose Donor Sperm: The Doctors Used Their Own." *New York Times*, August 21, 2019. https://www.nytimes.com/2019/08/21/health/sperm-donors-fraud-doctors.html.

Murphy-Sylla, Maybell. "Sperm Donor Kid." KQED, February 26, 2020. https://www.kqed.org/perspectives/201601139597/sperm-donor-kid.

National Conference of Commissioners on Uniform State Laws. "Uniform Parentage Act (2017)." 2017. https://www.uniformlaws.org/HigherLogic/System/DownloadDocumentFile.ashx?DocumentFileKey=e4a82c2a-f7cc-b33e-ed68-47ba88c36d92&forceDialog=0

NeJaime, Douglas. "The Nature of Parenthood." *Yale Law Journal* 126, no. 8 (2017): 2260–381.

Nelson, J. L. "Parental Obligations and the Ethics of Surrogacy: A Causal Perspective." *Public Affairs Quarterly* 5, no. 1 (January 1991): 49–61.

Nietzsche, Friedrich. *Beyond Good and Evil, Trans. R. J. Hollingdale*. London: Penguin (1973).

Nobes, Gavin, Georgia Panagiotaki, and Kenisha Russell Jonsson. "Child Homicides by Stepfathers: A Replication and Reassessment of the British Evidence." *Journal of Experimental Psychology: General* 148, no. 6 (June 2019): 1091–102.

Nordqvist, Petra, and Carol Smart. *Relative Strangers: Family Life, Genes and Donor Conception*. New York: Springer, 2014.

Nuffield Council on Bioethics. *Donor Conception: Ethical Aspects of Information Sharing*. London: Nuffield Council on Bioethics, 2013.

NW Cryobank. "Frequently Asked Questions about Using Donor Sperm." Accessed May 19, 2020. https://www.nwcryobank.com/donor-sperm-faqs/.

Obergefell v Hodges (135 S. Ct. 2584, 2600-01 (2015)

O'Donovan, Katherine. "'What Shall We Tell the Children?' Reflections on Children's Perspectives and the Reproduction Revolution." In *Birthrights: Law and Ethics at the Beginnings of Life*, edited by Robert Lee and Derek Morgan, 122–40. Routledge, 2003.

Ondaatje, Michael. *Warlight*. New York: Knopf Doubleday, 2018.

Oyserman, Daphna, Kristen Elmore, George Smith, Mark R. Leary, and June Price Tangney. "Self, Self-Concept and Identity." In *Handbook of Self and Identity*, edited by Mark R. Leary and June Price Tangney, 69–104. New York: Guilford Press, 2012.

Pacey, Allan. "Sperm Donor Recruitment in the UK." *Obstetrician & Gynaecologist* 12, no. 1 (2010): 43–48.

Passmore, N. L., A. R. Foulstone, and J. A. Feeney. "Openness and Secrecy in Adoptive Families and Possible Effects on the Interpersonal Relationships of Adult Adoptees." In *Relationships—Near and Far: Proceedings of the APS Psychology of Relationships Interest Group 6th Annual Conference* edited by Barry J. Fallon. Melbourne: Australian Psychological Society, 2006.

Paul, Laurie Ann. *Transformative Experience*. Oxford: Oxford University Press, 2014.

Paul, Laurie Ann. "What You Can't Expect When You're Expecting." *Res Philosophica* 92, no. 2 (2015): 149–70.

Paul, Marilyn S., and Roni Berger. "Topic Avoidance and Family Functioning in Families Conceived with Donor Insemination." *Human Reproduction* 22, no. 9 (September 1, 2007): 2566–71. https://doi.org/10.1093/humrep/dem174.

Pennings, Guido. "Disclosure of Donor Conception, Age of Disclosure and the Well-Being of Donor Offspring." *Human Reproduction* 32, no. 5 (May 1, 2017): 969–73.

The Personal Responsibility and Work Opportunity Reconciliation Act of 1996, Pub. L. No. 104–193, 110 STAT. 2105 (1996).

Pollack, Jonathan. "Would You Rather Not Exist?," *We Are Donor Conceived*, accessed January 5th, 2020, https://www.wearedonorconceived.com/personal-stories/would-you-rather-not-exist/

Prince William County Public Schools, *Family Life Education Grade 8 Health: Curriculum Objectives For Use In Mapping Family Life Education Instruction* August, 2009.

Prince William County Public Schools, *Family Life Education, Elementary School Objectives*, https://www.pwcs.edu/academics___programs/science___family_life_education/family_life_education. Accessed May, 2021.

Prusak, Bernard G. *Parental Obligations and Bioethics: The Duties of a Creator*. New York: Routledge, 2013.

Ravitsky, Vardit. "Autonomous Choice and the Right to Know One's Genetic Origins." *Hastings Center Report* 44, no. 2 (2014): 36–37.

Ravitsky, Vardit. "Knowing Where You Come From: The Rights of Donor-Conceived Individuals and the Meaning of Genetic Relatedness." *Minnesota Journal of Law, Science & Technology* 11 (2010): 665–84.

Rawls, John. *Justice as Fairness: A Restatement*. Cambridge, MA: Harvard University Press, 2001.

Rulli, Tina. "Preferring a Genetically-Related Child." *Journal of Moral Philosophy* 13, no. 6 (2016): 669–98.

Rushdie, Salman. *The Moor's Last Sigh*. New York: Random House, 2011.

Russell, Camisha A. *The Assisted Reproduction of Race*. Bloomington: Indiana University Press, 2018.

Russell v Pasik, 178 So. 3d 59–60 (Fla. Dist. Ct. App. 2015).

Satz, Debra. "Markets in Women's Reproductive Labor." *Philosophy & Public Affairs* 21, no. 2 (1992): 107–31.

Savulescu, Julian, and Guy Kahane. "The Moral Obligation to Create Children with the Best Chance of the Best Life." *Bioethics* 23, no. 5 (2009): 274–90.

Scheib, Joanna E., Maura Riordan, and Susan Rubin. "Choosing Identity-Release Sperm Donors: The Parents' Perspective 13–18 Years Later." *Human Reproduction* 18, no. 5 (2003): 1115–27.

Scheib, Joanna E., Alice Ruby, and Jean Benward. "Who Requests Their Sperm Donor's Identity? The First Ten Years of Information Releases to Adults with Open-Identity Donors." *Fertility and Sterility* 107, no. 2 (2017): 483–93.

Schneider, David M. *American Kinship: A Cultural Account*. Chicago: University of Chicago Press, 2014.

Schoeman, Ferdinand. "Rights of Children, Rights of Parents, and the Moral Basis of the Family." *Ethics* 91, no. 1 (October 1, 1980): 6–19. https://doi.org/10.1086/292199.

Schroeder, Mark. *Slaves of the Passions*. New York: Oxford University Press, 2007.

Schuetze, Christopher F. "Dutch Fertility Doctor Swapped Donors' Sperm with His, Lawsuit Claims." *New York Times*, May 15, 2017. https://www.nytimes.com/2017/05/15/world/europe/dutch-fertility-doctor-swapped-donors-sperm-with-his-lawsuit-claims.html.

Schuman, Olivia. "The Value of Genetic Ties as Ethical Justification for Banning Gamete Donor Anonymity." PhD dissertation, York University, 2020. https://yorkspace.library.yorku.ca/xmlui/handle/10315/37789.

Shapiro, Dani. *Inheritance: A Memoir of Genealogy, Paternity, and Love*. New York: Anchor, 2020.

Shields, Liam. "How Bad Can a Good Enough Parent Be?" *Canadian Journal of Philosophy* 46, no. 2 (2016): 163–82.

Shiffrin, Seana Valentine. "Wrongful Life, Procreative Responsibility, and the Significance of Harm." *Legal Theory* 5, no. 2 (1999): 117–48.

Silverberg, Cory. *What Makes a Baby*. New York: Seven Stories Press, 2013.

Smith, Matthew Noah. "The Importance of What They Care About." *Philosophical Studies* 165, no. 2 (September 1, 2013): 297–314. https://doi.org/10.1007/s11098-012-9929-0.

Sobel, David. Review of *Slaves of the Passions*, by Mark Schroeder. Notre Dame Philosophical Reviews, April 25, 2009. https://ndpr.nd.edu/news/slaves-of-the-passions/.

Tabacco Mar, Ria. "Opinion: My Kid Has 2 Moms. Why Did She Say She's Thankful for 'Mommy and Daddy'?" *New York Times*, November 21, 2018. https://www.nytimes.com/2018/11/21/opinion/children-thanksgiving-gratitude-gay.html.

This American Life. "Crunk in the Trunk." December 12, 2017. https://www.thisamericanlife.org/279/auto-show/act-one.

This American Life. "585: In Defense of Ignorance." December 14, 2017. https://www.thisamericanlife.org/585/transcript.

Tronto, Joan C. "The 'Nanny' Question in Feminism." *Hypatia* 17, no. 2 (2002): 34–51.

Turkmendag, Ilke. "It Is Just a 'Battery': 'Right' to Know in Mitochondrial Replacement." *Science, Technology, & Human Values* 43, no. 1 (January 1, 2018): 56–85.

Turkmendag, Ilke. "When Sperm Cannot Travel: Experiences of UK Would-Be Parents Seeking Treatment Abroad." In *European Law and New Health Technologies* edited by Flear, M.L., Farrell, A.M., Hervey, T.K., Murphy, T, 362–80. Oxford: Oxford University Press, 2013.

Turner, Amanda J., and Adrian Coyle. "What Does It Mean to Be a Donor Offspring? The Identity Experiences of Adults Conceived by Donor Insemination and the Implications for Counselling and Therapy." *Human Reproduction* 15, no. 9 (2000): 2041–51.

US Department of Health and Human Services. *AFCARS Report # 10*. June 30, 2006. https://www.acf.hhs.gov/cb/report/afcars-report-10.

Vanfraussen, Katrien, Ingrid Ponjaert-Kristoffersen, and Anne Brewaeys. "Why Do Children Want to Know More about the Donor? The Experience of Youngsters Raised in Lesbian Families." *Journal of Psychosomatic Obstetrics & Gynecology* 24, no. 1 (2003): 31–38.

Velleman, J. David. "Family History." *Philosophical Papers* 34, no. 3 (2005): 357–78.

Velleman, J. David. "The Gift of Life." *Philosophy & Public Affairs* 36, no. 3 (2008): 245–66.

Velleman, J. David. "III. Love and Nonexistence." *Philosophy & Public Affairs* 36, no. 3 (2008): 266–88.

We Are Donor Conceived. "Voices from the Offspring: Identity Formation." November 13, 2017. https://www.wearedonorconceived.com/personal-stories/voices-from-the-offspring-identity-formation/.

Walker, Iain, and Pia Broderick. "The Psychology of Assisted Reproduction—or Psychology Assisting Its Reproduction?" *Australian Psychologist* 34, no. 1 (1999): 38–44.

Weinberg, Rivka. *The Risk of a Lifetime: How, When, and Why Procreation May Be Permissible*. New York: Oxford University Press, 2016.

Witt, Charlotte. "Family Resemblances: Adoption, Personal Identity, and Genetic Essentialism." In *Adoption Matters: Philosophical and Feminist Essays*, edited by Sally Haslanger and Charlotte Witt, 265–90. Ithaca, NY: Cornell University Press, 2005.

Witt, Charlotte. "Family, Self and Society: A Critique of the Bionormative Conception of the Family." In *Family-Making: Contemporary Ethical Challenges*, edited by Carolyn MacLeod and Françoise Baylis, 49–63. Oxford University Press, 2014.

Wolf, Susan. *Meaning in Life and Why It Matters*. Princeton, NJ: Princeton University Press, 2012.

Wrigley, Anthony, Stephen Wilkinson, and John B. Appleby. "Mitochondrial Replacement: Ethics and Identity." *Bioethics* 29, no. 9 (2015): 631–38.

Yancy, George. "Opinion: Ahmaud Arbery and the Ghosts of Lynchings Past." *New York Times*, May 12, 2020. https://www.nytimes.com/2020/05/12/opinion/ahmaud-arbery-georgia-lynching.html.

Yoffe, Emily. "My Husband's Other Wife: She Died, So I Could Find the Man I Love." *Slate*, June 16, 2009. https://slate.com/human-interest/2009/06/my-husbands-other-wife-she-died-so-i-could-find-the-man-i-love.html.

Young, Iris Marion. *Justice and the Politics of Difference*. Princeton, NJ: Princeton University Press, 2011.

Index

For the benefit of digital users, indexed terms that span two pages (e.g., 52–53) may, on occasion, appear on only one of those pages.

Tables and figures are indicated by *t* and *f* following the page number